Self-Assessment Colour Review of

Gastroenterology

Alastair Forbes
BSc MD FRCP
St Mark's Hospital
Harrow, UK

Norman H Gilinsky
MD FACG
Division of Digestive Diseases
Department of Internal Medicine
University of Cincinnati College of Medicine, USA

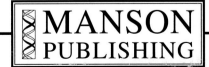

MANSON
PUBLISHING

Acknowledgements

We acknowledge the extreme patience of our contributors on both sides of the Atlantic during the editing and publishing phase of this project. Apart from those colleagues who provided questions, we would also like to thank those who contributed illustrative materials for this Review. Finally, we appreciate the ongoing encouragement of our respective wives, Laura and Stephanie.

AF, NHG

Copyright © 1999 Manson Publishing Ltd
ISBN 1-874545-47-2

For full details of all Manson Publishing titles, please write to:
Manson Publishing Ltd, 73 Corringham Road, London NW11 7DL, UK.

Design and layout: Judith Campbell.
Project management: John Ormiston.
Colour reproduction: Reed Digital, Ipswich, UK.
Printed by Grafos SA, Barcelona, Spain.

Preface

Physicians and other healthcare professionals are being increasingly overwhelmed by the demands of providing optimal patient care, while simultaneously endeavouring to keep current with developments in pathophysiology, molecular genetics, diagnostic techniques and therapeutics. Practitioners have to sift through a flood of information presented via journal articles, reference texts, symposia, as well as from audiocassettes, videotapes and Internet resources. This Review is intended to provide the reader with an overview of the subject by means of illustrated case histories, in the belief that this format is most productive in terms of readability and education. To accommodate as much data as space and budget would allow, we have attempted to present the material in a succinct yet readable Question and Answer style. Although the UK and US healthcare systems (and spelling!) are very different, we were pleasantly surprised with respect to the similarity in the spectrum of disorders encountered and clinical approach employed by our respective contributors. While we do not expect every clinician to manage all the clinical problems presented here in a similar manner, we hope that the reader will find this Review a worthwhile and educational tool.

AF, NHG

Contributors

John Baillie, MB, ChB, FRCP (Glasg.), Duke University Medical Center, Durham, North Carolina, USA

Oliver Cass, MD, Hennepin City Medical Center, Minneapolis, Minnesota, USA

David Casson, MD, MRCP, Royal Free Hospital, London, UK

Umakant Dave, MD, MRCP, St Andrew's Hospital, Billericay, UK

Anton Emmanuel, MB, MRCP, St Mark's Hospital, Harrow, UK

Alastair Forbes, BSc, MD, FRCP, St Mark's Hospital, Harrow, UK

Bahram Forouzandeh, MD, University of Louisville, Louisville, Kentucky, USA

Norman H Gilinsky, MD, MRCP (UK), FACG, University of Cincinnati Medical Center, Cincinnati, Ohio, USA

Adam Harris, MD, MRCP, Kent and Sussex Hospital, Tunbridge Wells, UK

Timothy Heyman, MB, MBA, MRCP, Kingston Hospital, Kingston-upon-Thames, UK

Bret Lashner, MD, Cleveland Clinic Foundation, Cleveland, Ohio, USA

Edward V Loftus Jr., MD , Mayo Clinic, Rochester, Minnesota, USA

Steven Mann, MB, MRCP, St Mark's Hospital, Harrow, UK

John Martin, MB, MRCP, St Mark's Hospital, Harrow, UK

Stephen P Martin, MD, University of Cincinnati Medical Center, Cincinnati, Ohio, USA

Craig J McClain, MD, University of Kentucky Medical Center, Lexington, Kentucky, USA

David C Metz, MD, University of Pennsylvania, Philadelphia, Pennsylvania, USA

Andrew Millar, MD, MRCP, North Middlesex Hospital, London, UK

Magda Newton, MD, MRCP, Oldchurch Hospital, Romford, UK

Chai Li Ng, MB, MRCP, Negeri Sembilan, Malaysia

Satish SC Rao, MD, PhD, University of Iowa, Iowa City, Iowa, USA

Colin Rudolph, MD, Children's Hospital Medical Center, Cincinnati, Ohio, USA

Bradley Shapiro, MD, Cleveland Clinic Foundation, Cleveland, Ohio, USA

Christopher Sheen, MB, MRCP, Southampton General Hospital, Southampton, UK

Kate Tonge, MB, MRCP, St Mark's Hospital, Harrow, UK

Andrew Veitch, MD, MRCP, Royal London Hospital, London, UK

Robert Weesner, MD, Veterans Administration Medical Center, Cincinnati, Ohio, USA

David C Wolf, MD, New York Medical College, Valhalla, New York, USA

Abbreviations

AFP	Alpha-fetoprotein	INR	International normalized ratio
AIDS	Acquired immunodeficiency syndrome	JVD	Jugulovenous distension
		JVP	Jugular venous pressure
ALA	Aminolaevulinic acid	KS	Kaposi's sarcoma
ALP	Alkaline phosphatase	LFT	Liver function tests
ALT	Alanine aminotransferase	LOS	Lower oesophageal sphincter
ANA	Anti-nuclear antibody	MAI	*Mycobacterium avium-intracellulare*
5-ASA	5-Aminosalicylic acid	MALToma	Mucosa-associated lymphoid tissue tumour
AST	Aspartate aminotransferase		
BUN	Blood urea nitrogen	MCH	Mean corpuscular haemoglobin
CCK	Cholecystokinin	MCV	Mean corpuscular volume
CEA	Carcinoembryonic antigen	MEN	Multiple endocrine neoplasia
CHRPE	Congenital hypertrophy of the retinal pigment epithelium	MRI	Magnetic resonance imaging
		NG	Nasogastric
CIIP	Chronic idiopathic intestinal pseudo-obstruction	NLH	Nodular lymphoid hyperplasia
		NSAID	Non-steroidal anti-inflammatory drug
CMSE	Cows' milk-sensitive enteropathy		
CMV	Cytomegalovirus	NUD	Non-ulcer dyspepsia
CNS	Central nervous system	OGD	Oesophagogastroduodenoscopy
COAD	Chronic obstructive airways disease	PA	Pernicious anaemia
COPD	Chronic obstructive pulmonary disease	PAS	Periodic acid–Schiff
		PBG	Porphobilinogen
CRP	C-reactive protein	PCR	Polymerase chain reaction
CREST	Calcinosis, Raynaud's, (o)esophageal involvement, sclerodactyly, telangiectasia	PEG	Percutaneous endoscopic gastrostomy
		PEJ	Percutaneous endoscopic jejunostomy
CT	Computed tomography		
CVS	Cyclical vomiting syndrome	PET	Positron emission tomography
DALM	Dysplasia-associated lesion or mass	PG	Pyoderma gangrenosum
ECG	Electrocardiogram	PMC	Pseudomembranous colitis
ECL	Enterochromaffin-like cell	PSC	Primary sclerosing cholangitis
EGE	Eosinophilic gastroenteritis	PT	Prothrombin time
EHEC	Enterohaemorrhagic *E. coli*	PTT	Partial thromboplastin time
ELISA	Enzyme-linked immunosorbent assay	RDA	Recommended daily allowance
		SGOT	Serum glutamic-oxaloacetic transaminase (or AST)
ERCP	Endoscopic retrograde cholangiopancreatography	SGPT	Serum glutamate-pyruvate transaminase (or AST)
ESR	Erythrocyte sedimentation rate		
ETEC	Enterotoxigenic *Escherichia coli*	SIADH	Syndrome of inappropriate anti-diuretic hormone generation
FAP	Familial adenomatous polyposis		
FBC	Full blood count	SLE	Systemic lupus erythematosus
FDG	Fluoro-deoxyglucose	SMA	Superior mesenteric artery
5-FU	5-Fluorouracil	SRUS	Solitary rectal ulcer syndrome
GALT	Gut-associated lymphoid tissue	SSA	Sjögren's syndrome antibody
GI	Gastrointestinal	TB	Tuberculosis
GIP	Gastrin inhibitory peptide	TIBC	Total iron-binding capacity
GORD	Gastro-oesophageal reflux disease	TIPS	Transjugular intrahepatic portosystemic shunt
GRP	Gastrin-releasing peptide		
H2R	H2 receptor	TNF	Tumour necrosis factor
HCP	Hereditary coproporphyria	TPN	Total parenteral nutrition
5-HIAA	5-Hydroxyindole acetic acid	TSH	Thyroid-stimulating hormone
HIV	Human immunodeficiency virus	U & E	Urea and electrolytes
HP	*Helicobacter pylori*	VIP	Vasoactive intestinal peptide
IBD	Inflammatory bowel disease	VP	Variegate porphyria
IF	Intrinsic factor	WBC	White blood cell
IL-1	Interleukin-1	ZES	Zollinger–Ellison syndrome

1 A 16-year-old female presents with a 3-month history of the passage of blood and mucus per rectum, anal itch and discomfort, and a sense of incomplete evacuation. A long-standing history of constipation continues despite drinking prune juice. There is no loss of appetite or weight, and abdominal examination is normal. She denies any digital manipulation or trauma. Rectal examination reveals somewhat reduced tone, and an indurated area is palpable anteriorly in the rectum.
Excessive perineal descent is demonstrated when she is asked to bear down. A sigmoidoscopy demonstrates a 2 cm, shallow, ulcerated area with a rim of oedematous, erythematous mucosa 4 cm inside the rectum (1).

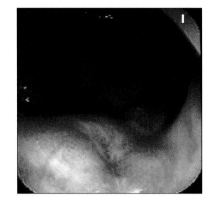

i. What is the likely diagnosis?
ii. Discuss the aetiology.
iii. What is histology likely to demonstrate?
iv. Describe treatment modalities.
v. What complications may occur?

2 A full-term 3.5 kg baby born after an uncomplicated pregnancy is breast-fed after birth. On day 2 of life, watery bowel movements and a distended abdomen are noted. Breast-feeding is discontinued and a cow's milk-based formula is begun. By day 7 of life, the infant is noted to have marked abdominal distention with ascitic fluid, profuse diarrhoea and peripheral oedema. The stool is watery but contains no occult blood. Laboratory values include: haemoglobin 13.0 g/dl, WBC count $11.5 \times 10^9/l$ (11 500/mm^3) (with 90% neutrophils, 5% lymphocytes, 2% eosinophils), SGOT (AST) 35 u/l, SGPT (ALT) 44 u/l, total bilirubin 41 μmol/l (2.4 mg/dl) and albumin 18 g/l. Urinalysis is normal. A barium study is performed (2a).

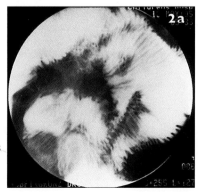

i. What is the cause of the hypoalbuminaemia?
ii. Which confirmatory diagnostic test should be performed?
iii. Discuss the likely aetiology.
iv. Describe the type of ascites likely in this case.
v. Discuss treatment of this disorder.

1 i. Solitary rectal ulcer syndrome (SRUS). Rectal prolapse, factitious trauma, infections, neoplastic lesions, prolapsing haemorrhoids and inflammatory bowel disease are possible.

ii. SRUS probably does not have a single cause. The rectal mucosa may be ischaemic as a result of traction and pressure from an over-reactive puborectalis, and from anterior rectal wall prolapse associated with excessive perineal descent. However, prolapse cannot always be demonstrated in cases of this type.

iii. Histology demonstrates obliteration of the lamina propria by fibromuscular proliferation of the muscularis mucosae, which becomes thickened and extends between the crypts, and a diffuse increase in mucosal collagen.

iv. A high-fibre diet and avoidance of straining at stool help to ease symptoms. Rectopexy may be necessary for those with associated rectal prolapse. Ensuring a regular bowel action, excluding obstructive defaecation and retraining, with biofeedback techniques, constitutes a good approach.

v. Complications such as blood loss and stricturing are rare. Depression and behaviour disorders are common.

2 i. Protein-losing enteropathy.

ii. Protein in the stool may be confirmed by an elevated faecal alpha-1-antitrypsin.

iii. Rotavirus or other enteric viruses may result in severe mucosal atrophy with biopsies indistinguishable from coeliac disease. *Giardia lamblia* is uncommon in the immediate perinatal period. Structural disorders of the lymphatic vessels may also result in intestinal leakage of protein. In this infant, the associated hypolipidaemia and lymphopenia suggests lymphangiectasia.

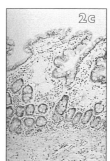

Confirmation of the diagnosis requires small-bowel biopsy. Snowflake-like lesions which result from the lacteals being dilated and filled with fat are observed endoscopically or on gross biopsy specimens (**2b**). Dilated empty lymphatic vessels are evident in the small-bowel biopsy (**2c**; standard haematoxylin and eosin staining). Frozen section with oil red O stain more clearly demonstrates the lesion (**2d**).

iv. Paracentesis of the ascitic fluid may reveal transudative or chylous fluid.

v. Treatment limits in-take of long-chain fats to decrease the amount of villous lymphatic distention. Calories are provided as medium-chain triglycerides. Supplementation with fat-soluble vitamins is usually required. Occasionally, intravenous lipid is needed to provide essential fatty acids.

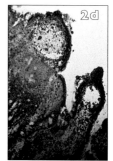

3 A 47-year-old man presented with a 48-hour history of fresh haematemesis and passing black stool.
i. What specific questions would you wish to ask?
ii. What information could be gained from the initial examination?
iii. How would you manage this patient?
iv. What is the lesion shown in the stomach (3)?

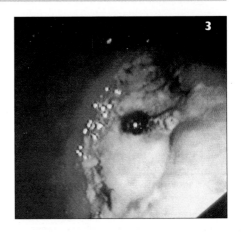

4 A 45-year-old woman patient presented to the outpatient clinic complaining of intermittent, dull abdominal discomfort and an odd sensation which altered position as she moved. She was otherwise fit and examination was unremarkable. Ultrasound scanning of the gallbladder was normal and endoscopy was then performed.
i. What is seen in 4?
ii. What could be the constituents of the abnormality?
iii. What treatment is available?

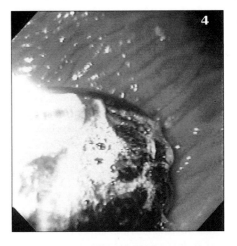

5 A 55-year-old man required three admissions to hospital over the past year with abdominal pain.
i. Comment on the radiographic findings (5).
ii. What is the diagnosis?
iii. What is the most common aetiology?
iv. What complications may occur as a result of this condition?
v. What are the therapeutic options?

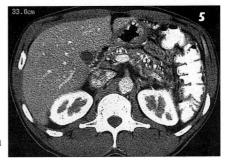

3–5: Answers

3 i. A past history of peptic ulcer or liver disease, ingestion of NSAIDs and iron therapy are sought. Other features which may help include symptoms suggestive of a bleeding diathesis, symptomatic anaemia and evidence of shock.
ii. Shock (rapid pulse and postural hypotension), clinical anaemia, and melaena indicate the severity of a gastrointestinal bleed. Bruising or petechiae suggests a clotting disorder or platelet dysfunction, and there may be signs of chronic liver disease.
iii. The patient is resuscitated with whole blood; a central line is inserted to assess fluid replacement if the patient is hypotensive. Admission to a unit experienced in the management of acute gastrointestinal bleeding is recommended. Early endoscopy defines the cause of the bleeding and often allows therapeutic intervention. Surgeons are informed of the patient's admission.
iv. An ulcer with a visible vessel in its base that requires immediate therapy.

4 i. This is a gastric bezoar.
ii. Bezoars are foreign matter concretions. They occur rarely and may be found incidentally. They are more common with anatomic abnormalities of the gut, either developmental or iatrogenic, and can comprise a variety of constituents such as hair (trichobezoars), vegetable matter (phytobezoars), ingested foreign matter (e.g. cement), medication (e.g. aluminium hydroxide concretions in patients with renal failure), or fungi. They occur when foreign matter is unable to leave the stomach due to size, outlet obstruction, motility disorders or congenital pyloric stenosis.

Patients are often asymptomatic or present with vague symptoms. Acute presentation, with abdominal bloating and vomiting and signs of obstruction, rarely occurs.

Investigations include plain abdominal radiographs, barium studies or endoscopy.
iii. Dissolution of the bezoar with enzymes is useful to digest the protein, cellulose and mucous components of phytobezoars. Other bezoars may need to be removed endoscopically (if small enough), by fragmentation, or by open surgical operation, particularly if complications such as obstruction have occurred.

5 i. This is a CT scan showing an atrophic pancreas with dilatation of the pancreatic duct and calcification within the body.
ii. Chronic calcific pancreatitis.
iii. Chronic alcohol excess, the most common cause of chronic pancreatitis, accounting for over 70% of cases in most countries. Other causes of acute pancreatitis rarely progress to chronic damage.
iv. Progressive loss of the exocrine and (to a lesser extent) the endocrine gland leads to pancreatic insufficiency and diabetes. Oedema of the pancreatic head occasionally causes obstructive jaundice; this is more common in pancreatic carcinoma, which is a potential complication of chronic pancreatitis.
v. Therapeutic options are limited, but include strong advice to abstain from alcohol. Analgesia may require opiates, transcutaneous nerve simulators, or coeliac plexus nerve block. In exocrine insufficiency, pancreatic enzyme supplements are required and may also ease the pain. Stenting of the pancreatic duct or surgical drainage (pancreato-jejunostomy) may help if there is significant pancreatic duct obstruction.

6 A thin, 17-year-old Irish girl has had diarrhoea
with pale offensive stools for 6 months.
i. Comment on the barium follow-through
examination (6).
ii. What is the most likely diagnosis?
iii. What confirmatory investigations would be
most helpful?
iv. What are the long-term complications of this
condition?

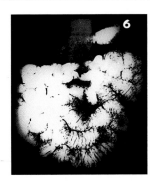

7 A 21-year-old man had
presented some years earlier
with recurrent abdominal
pain and diarrhoea.
i. What do the height (7a)
and weight (7b) charts
demonstrate?
ii. What does his recent
bone radiograph show (7c)?
iii. What radiological
diagnosis is suggested by
the small-bowel films (7d)?
iv. What findings in the
rectal biopsy (7e) lead to a confident
diagnosis?

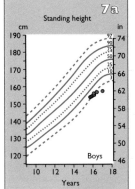

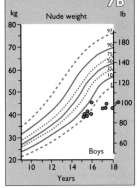

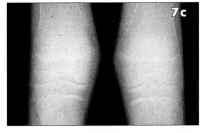

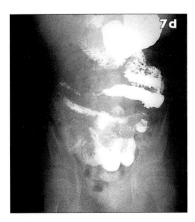

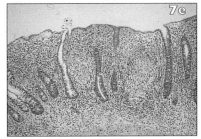

6 i. There are dilated jejunal loops with thickened folds and flocculation of barium.
ii. Coeliac disease. The prevalence varies, but is highest in the west of Ireland where it is 1 in 300. Diarrhoea, flatulence, weight loss and lethargy may not be prominent.
iii. Duodenal biopsy. Barium follow-through is not specific. Biopsy confirms sub-total villous atrophy with crypt hyperplasia, increased inflammatory infiltrate and increased intra-epithelial lymphocytes. Serum anti-endomysial antibody is currently the most sensitive and specific serum marker for coeliac disease, and disappears following response to a strict gluten-free diet.
iv. Untreated severe coeliac disease eventually results in vitamin deficiencies due to malabsorption and may present with tetany (vitamin-D deficiency), haemorrhage (vitamin-K deficiency) or peripheral neuropathy (vitamin-B_{12} deficiency). An increased risk of gastrointestinal and non-gastrointestinal malignancies should be considered and excluded in relapse after initial response to a gluten-free diet.

7 i. Growth retardation.
ii. Failure of epiphyseal fusion.
iii. Extensive small-bowel Crohn's disease.
iv. The presence of a granuloma, and a transmural chronic inflammatory infiltrate.
   Approximately 20% of Crohn's disease presents before the age of 20 years. The anatomic distribution of disease is similar to that in adults. Approximately 15% of children have perianal disease. The clinical manifestations are similar to those of adults, with the addition of growth failure which may precede overt GI symptoms by years.
   Growth failure can be defined as: cessation of linear growth for more than 6 months; decrease of one standard deviation in height centile; a bone age delay of more than 2 years. The prevalence of growth failure in children and adolescents with Crohn's disease is approximately 30%.
   It is important to differentiate growth retardation from genetic short stature or constitutionally delayed growth, and heights and weights must be tabulated over time. Normally, a growing child maintains a constant relationship to the centile lines, and rarely crosses a line. Those with genetic or constitutional short stature have growth curves parallel to those of normal children (i.e. normal height velocity). In children with disease-related growth problems, reduction or cessation of height velocity occurs.
   Radiological bone age helps to distinguish genetic short stature from growth retardation due to disease, as genetically short children have bone age corresponding to chronological age, but the growth retarded have bone age less than chronological age.
   Growth retardation is of multifactorial origin:
(a) Reduced nutrient intake: post-prandial pain or diarrhoea; altered taste sensation (e.g. zinc deficiency and metronidazole use); early satiety (delayed gastric emptying).
(b) Malabsorption: loss of surface area because of disease or resection; bacterial overgrowth.
(c) Increased losses: bleeding; protein-losing enteropathy; fistulas.
(d) Drugs which interfere with metabolism such as: sulphasalazine (folate); cholestyramine (fat and fat-soluble vitamins).
(e) Increased demands: sepsis and fever; increased cell turnover and demands of rapid growth; replacement of losses.

8 A 57-year-old man with a 17-year history of ulcerative colitis which was usually well controlled presented with bloody, formed stools and rapid weight loss over about 6 weeks. Examination was unremarkable and at rigid sigmoidoscopy the colitis appeared quiescent. A barium enema was arranged (8).

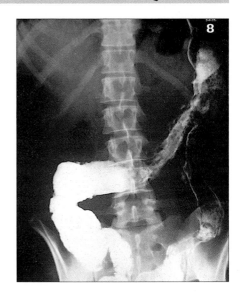

i. Describe what is seen
ii. Was this avoidable?

9 A 31-year-old man with AIDS complains of upper abdominal pain, weight loss and soft stools without blood for the past 6 weeks. He has a history of viral hepatitis, fungal oesophagitis, cytomegalovirus retinitis and *Pneumocystis carinii* pneumonia, and is on appropriate prophylaxis at the present time. He is not known to have peptic ulcer disease and does not use ulcerogenic medications. Physical examination is remarkable for muscular wasting and upper abdominal tenderness. Rectal examination is unremarkable. His last CD4+ lymphocyte count was 10/ml (normal, >500/ml). There is a mild pancytopenia. The serum amylase is normal. There is no faecal leukocytosis, but occult blood is present. Cultures and a variety of special stains fail to reveal any pathogens. An upper endoscopy reveals violaceous lesions in the duodenum (9a).

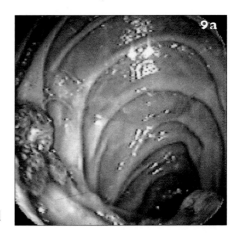

i. What is the probable diagnosis?
ii. How may this be confirmed?
iii. Comment on non-AIDS populations who may be at-risk for this disorder.
iv. Discuss presentation and treatment of this disorder.
v. Comment on other gastrointestinal malignancies in patients with AIDS.

8 & 9: Answers

8 i. The classic 'hose-pipe' of chronic ulcerative colitis on the left and a narrowed, irregular area proximal to the splenic flexure which is an adenocarcinoma.
ii. There is an increased risk of colorectal carcinoma in long-standing extensive colitis, and many recommend surveillance colonoscopy for disease proximal to the splenic flexure of more than 10 years' duration. Although there are good supportive data, there have been no controlled evaluations of surveillance. The aim is to detect early curable cancers and pre-invasive dysplasia. High-grade dysplasia is associated with colonoscopically inapparent carcinoma in up to one-third of cases and can be expected to progress to this rapidly in the remainder without colectomy. Low-grade dysplasia often progresses to high-grade dysplasia or carcinoma (50% within 3 years). It is probably wise to advise colectomy. If dysplasia is demonstrated in association with a macroscopic lesion – the so-called DALM – then colectomy is always indicated.

9 i. Violaceous, flat macular or nodular lesions with a bosselated surface suggest Kaposi's sarcoma (KS). It occurs mainly in homosexual men with AIDS.

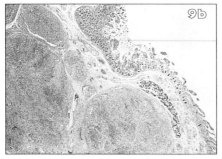

ii. Biopsy (**9b**) generally confirms the diagnosis, but superficial specimens may not allow detection of the characteristic erythrocyte-trapping spindle cells. Large biopsy forceps are therefore advised. The lesions are generally multifocal and visceral involvement is extensive. Once diagnosed, gastrointestinal work-up is unlikely to be useful.
iii. Before AIDS, 'classic' Kaposi's sarcoma was endemic in Africa, involving the lower extremities of elderly individuals. This has a far better prognosis than KS in the immunocompromised.
iv. Most patients with KS have cutaneous or oropharyngeal lesions, but a gastrointestinal presentation may be its first sign. The majority of lesions are clinically silent, but pain, ulceration, haemorrhage, obstruction and perforation may occur. Treatment is generally reserved for symptomatic lesions. Prognosis is poor and treatment does not prevent progression of AIDS. KS lesions tend to be sensitive to chemotherapy and radiation, and up to 50% respond to alpha-interferon. Surgery may be necessary for intestinal obstruction, perforation or intractable haemorrhage.
v. Loss of immune surveillance as a result of T-cell deficiency promotes malignant lymphoproliferation in AIDS. Non-Hodgkin B-cell lymphomas are common. Highly aggressive tumours involve the stomach, anorectum and liver predominantly. T-cell lymphomas are associated with the human T-lymphotropic virus type I. Carcinoma of the anorectum is also seen.

10 Shown in 10 is the colon of a 74-year-old woman undergoing colonoscopy as part of a series of investigations for iron-deficiency anaemia.
i. What is the diagnosis?
ii. Outline the pathogenesis of this condition.
iii. What complications may arise, and what is their differential diagnosis?
iv. What treatment should be recommended to this woman?

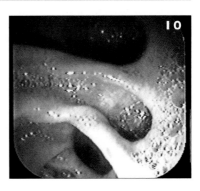

11 Shown in 11 is the endoscopic appearance of the caecum in a 42-year-old Asian woman who described lethargy ever since a visit to Bombay 2 months earlier. On further questioning, she also described mild central abdominal discomfort. Examination was normal apart from moderate pallor. Other investigations revealed: haemoglobin 9.2 g/dl; MCV 62 fl; leukocytes 4.3×10^9/l; eosinophils 10%; platelets 230×10^9/l; ESR 3 mm/h; renal and hepatic biochemistry normal; serum iron 4 µg/l; TIBC 85%. The upper gastrointestinal endoscopy was normal.
i. What are the abnormal findings?
ii. Could these explain the anaemia?
iii. What therapy is advised?

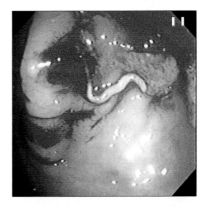

12 A 24-year-old male had a 10-year history of Crohn's disease (12). Colonoscopy was performed because of increasing, colicky pain affecting the left side of the abdomen and associated with abdominal distention.
i. What is the abnormality?
ii. What treatment is recommended?

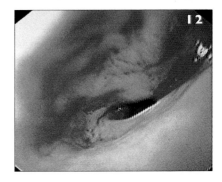
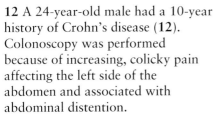

10–12: Answers

10 i. There is marked colonic diverticular disease.
ii. Colonic diverticula are thought to arise as a result of long-standing dietary fibre insufficiency. Small-volume stools require high intracolonic pressure for propulsion, and over many years this high pressure produces protrusion of the mucous membrane through the weaker points in the bowel wall (usually where vessels penetrate between the mesenteric border and the lateral taenia coli). The incidence of diverticular disease increases with age, and parallels a decrease in the tensile strength of both the longitudinal and circular muscle fibre layers. Colonic collagen becomes cross-linked after the age of 40, increasing colonic rigidity. Patients with primary collagen disorders, e.g. Ehlers–Danlos and Marfan's syndromes, develop diverticula at a much earlier age.
iii. The patient may develop diverticulitis; diverticular abscess; fistulae to other sites in the bowel, the bladder and the vagina; or peritonitis if free perforation into the peritoneum occurs. All are rare. Still less common are hydronephrosis from ureteric obstruction by a diverticular mass, and portal pyaemia with secondary liver abscess. The differential diagnosis for each of these complications is usually colorectal carcinoma or Crohn's disease. Diverticula may bleed slowly with resultant iron-deficiency anaemia, but more often bleeding presents acutely with major rectal haemorrhage. The differential diagnosis then is wider and includes inflammatory and ischaemic colitis and malignancy, but also angiodysplasia, telangiectasia, haemangioma, aorto-enteric fistula, and, of course, haemorrhoids!
iv. This woman is encouraged to increase her dietary fibre intake. A satisfactory clinical response can be expected in patients such as this by daily consumption of both bran and fruit.

11 i. The woman has a caecal worm. The macroscopic appearance (**11**) suggests that this is *Trichuris trichiura*, the whipworm. Infestation is endemic in many parts of the world and is often asymptomatic.
ii. Heavy infestations cause eosinophilia and may cause a mucosal infiltrate in the colon which can be friable and bleed. Although alternative explanations for the anaemia were correctly in this patient, none was found apart from moderate menorrhagia.
iii. A course of mebendazole and short-term iron supplementation.

12 i. There is a smooth stricture with little associated inflammation (**12**).
ii. It is worth considering therapy with mesalamine (mesalazine) and/or steroids, but these are unlikely to be effective in this case given the virtual absence of associated inflammation and an absence of an acute phase response. White cell scanning can help here, as it usually is normal if the main problem is fibrous stricturing, and a mechanical solution is required. The intervention of choice when there have been previous resections, and especially when small-bowel length is prejudiced, is stricturoplasty, or an even less invasive treatment using 'through the scope' balloons at colonoscopy.

13 Answer TRUE or FALSE to each of the following statements regarding pancreatic physiology.
i. Pain sensation from the pancreas travels to the brain via sympathetic afferent nerves.
ii. The endocrine portion of the pancreas comprises 2% of the total mass of the pancreas.
iii. The functional units of the exocrine pancreas are the islets of Langerhans.
iv. Pancreatic acinar cells secrete a fluid composed of sodium chloride and enzymes, whereas the duct cells (tubules) secrete fluid containing a high concentration of bicarbonate.
v. The concentration of bicarbonate varies with the flow rate of secretions.
vi. Steatorrhoea occurs when the pancreatic exocrine capacity is reduced by >20%.

14 A 76-year-old man is admitted with pneumonia. He has a history of cerebrovascular accidents and dementia and has been admitted on five occasions during the previous 12 months for pneumonic illnesses. His nurse reports that he requires assistance with feeding, which takes a long time to accomplish. He coughs frequently during and after feeds. An upper endoscopy performed 6 months previously following possible dysphagia, demonstrated a small hiatus hernia without stricturing. The patient appears wasted. He has pneumonic consolidation. The abdomen has no abnormality to palpation. A barium study to evaluate his swallowing function reveals spillover into the bronchial tree. The oesophagus appears normal.
i. What is the probable cause of his recurrent respiratory infections?
ii. Comment on his nutritional status.
iii. The family agree that no further investigations are indicated and treatment should be supportive only. Which methods of nutrient delivery are appropriate for this man?
iv. What are the complications of the nutrition delivery method utilized in **14a** and **14b**?
v. Comment on the influence of duodenal tube placement on the risk of future pneumonic episodes.

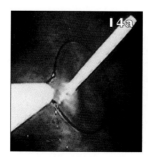
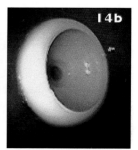

13 & 14: Answers

13 i. True. Extrinsic innervation of the pancreas is by the splanchnic and vagus nerves and consists of afferent sensory fibres and efferent secretory and vasomotor fibres. Intrinsic innervation consists of afferent sensory fibres, efferent parasympathetic pre- and post-ganglionic fibres, efferent sympathetic post-ganglionic fibres from the coeliac, mesenteric and other ganglia, and peptidergic fibres. There are pain receptors whose stimuli travel along sympathetic afferents to the brain.
ii. True. The exocrine pancreas comprises 85% of the total mass (80 g); the endocrine portion comprises 2% or less. The remainder is made up of connective tissue, nerves and blood vessels.
iii. False. The functional unit of the exocrine pancreas is the *acinus* and its associated *ductule*.
iv. True. Exocrine pancreatic secretion is composed of an enzyme-rich fluid produced by the acinar cells and a bicarbonate-rich fluid produced by the duct cells.
v. True. The flow rate of secretions through the pancreatic ducts varies from zero to 4 ml/min. As the rate increases, the concentrations of chloride and bicarbonate change reciprocally: chloride concentration falls and bicarbonate increases. Protein concentrations are higher in the basal state than in stimulated secretions. The concentrations of sodium and potassium appear to be independent of flow rate.
vi. False. Pancreatic enzymes are very efficient in promoting digestion of dietary fat. Studies have demonstrated that the functional capacity of the pancreas must be reduced by almost 90% before an excess of dietary fat appears in the stool.

14 i. Recurrent respiratory infections in cerebrovascular disease suggests aspiration. The neurological disorder results in transfer dysphagia. The previous endoscopy and current barium study effectively exclude significant oesophageal stricture or structural problem.
ii. The weight loss and wasting indicate suboptimal nutrition.
iii. These include nasogastric tube, nasoenteral tube and gastrostomy. Total parenteral nutrition is impractical and unnecessary.
iv. An intragastric view of a PEG device insertion is shown in **14a**; its internal bolster is shown in **14b**. Potential complications relate to the endoscopy, ileus, infection at the gastrostomy site, malplacement (perforation of contiguous organs), migration of the device (distally to obstruct the gastric outlet, or proximally to become 'buried' subcutaneously), bleeding (as a result of erosion of adjacent gastric mucosa), aspiration due to overdistention of the stomach, tube blockage due to concretions, failure to flush the tubing adequately following feeds or inappropriate placement of medications into the tubing.
v. Intragastric feeding may aggravate a tendency to reflux, particularly if the stomach is overdistended or if the patient remains horizontal during and following feeds. PEG feeding will not prevent aspiration of saliva. The PEG may be adapted to allow infusion into the distal duodenum/jejunum in patients who have delayed gastric emptying, structural abnormalities of the gastric outlet or recurrent vomiting in the absence of intestinal obstruction, but a reduced frequency of aspiration has not yet been confirmed.

15 A 22-year-old woman presents with a 4-month history of right lower quadrant abdominal pain, a 9 kg (20 lb) weight loss, and intermittent diarrhoea. A flexible sigmoidoscopy to 60 cm fails to reveal any mucosal abnormality. A small-bowel radiograph was requested (15).

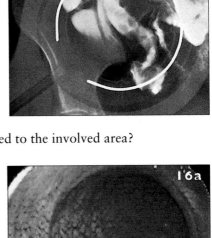

i. What is the most likely diagnosis?
ii. What is the differential diagnosis?
iii. What further investigations should be undertaken?
iv. What is the initial treatment recommendation?
v. What complications could occur related to the involved area?

16 Endoscopic views are shown (16a and 16b) of the distal duodenum in separate patients who have a similar clinical presentation. Both complain of chronic diarrhoea with weight loss (persistent over the preceding few months) and abdominal bloating with occasional nausea. Abdominal examination is unremarkable, and the faecal fat stain is positive in both. The endoscopist describes the mucosal fold pattern in 16a as featureless, while that in 16b is uniformly nodular.

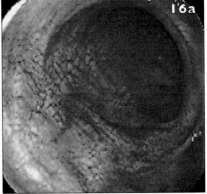

i. Which diagnoses are suggested in each case?
ii. Which additional studies may be indicated?
iii. Which disease associations may be present?
iv. How should the diarrhoea be treated?
v. What additional complications may occur, common to both entities?

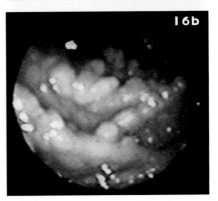

15 i. Luminal narrowing in the terminal ileum with an irregular mucosal pattern suggests ulceration. There is separation of contiguous bowel loops. These findings are characteristic of the lesions of Crohn's disease. This patient is likely to have a tender, right lower quadrant mass.
ii. Other diseases that should be considered include intestinal lymphoma, tuberculosis, and *Yersinia* infection.
iii. A colonoscopy with biopsies of the terminal ileum should confirm the diagnosis of Crohn's disease. Stool cultures help to rule out *Yersinia enterocolitica*.
iv. Initial treatment with corticosteroids and/or mesalamine (mesalazine) is tried. If ineffective or if symptoms recur following taper of steroids, resection is considered.
v. Obstruction due to an inflammatory or fibrotic stricture, fistulation, perforation, malabsorption of bile salts and vitamin B_{12}.

16 i. A flat mucosa is an endoscopic feature of coeliac disease, but also occurs in scleroderma and Zollinger–Ellison syndrome. A uniformly nodular pattern is observed in immunodeficiency states, particularly nodular lymphoid hyperplasia (NLH), agammaglobulinaemia, lymphoma, alpha chain disease, amyloidosis and infection with *Mycobacterium avium* complex.
ii. An endoscopic biopsy is examined for the presence of villous atrophy and other features of coeliac disease (**16c**), submucosal lymphocyte aggregations (NLH) and *Giardia*. Antigliadin and antiendomysial antibodies may be positive in coeliac disease. Serum IgA and IgM deficiencies may be associated with NLH.
iii. Patients with coeliac disease should undergo a nutritional workup. NLH is seen in immunodeficiency states, especially IgA deficiency states. Patients with IgA deficiency are essentially healthy but predisposed to developing giardiasis. Numerous stool examinations may be necessary to identify it, including immunoprecipitation assay of the stool for *Giardia* antigens and small-bowel biopsy.
iv. Patients with coeliac disease must be placed on a strict gluten-free diet. Poor compliance or the possibility of collagenous sprue should be considered in patients whose response is suboptimal. A thorough search for *Giardia* is made in patients with NLH. Otherwise, symptomatic treatment with antidiarrhoeals or treatment for bacterial overgrowth may be prudent.

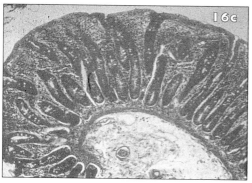

v. Patients with coeliac disease as well as NLH are prone to the development of lymphomas, which must be considered when symptoms persist despite treatment, or a small-bowel barium study demonstrates deformity. Steatorrhoea may occur in both diseases. Both may unmask a latent lactose intolerance.

17 A 60-year-old woman notes rectal bleeding and pain with defecation for 4 months. Digital rectal examination reveals a firm, irregular mass at the anal verge, and flexible sigmoidoscopy (retroflexed in the rectum to view the squamocolumnar junction) reveals the lesion seen in 17. Biopsies demonstrate a well-differentiated squamous cell carcinoma.

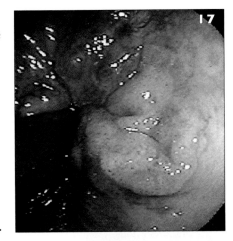

i. What is the nature of the lesion demonstrated?
ii. How may the diagnosis be confirmed?
iii. Which risk factors have been associated with this lesion?
iv. Comment on the route of progression of this lesion.
v. Comment on treatment modalities.

18 A 60-year-old man has had recurrent episodes of transient itching and jaundice for 4 months. At ERCP, the duodenal papilla has been replaced by an irregular, friable mass (18a). The cholangiogram (18b) and pancreatogram both demonstrate gross obstruction at the level of the papilla. Endoscopic biopsies reveal adenomatous tissue without evidence of malignancy.

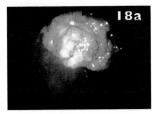

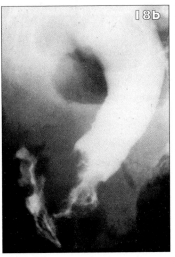

i. Comment on the benign nature of the biopsy findings.
ii. Discuss the prognosis of ampullary cancer versus ductal adenocarcinoma of the pancreas.
iii. Discuss the role of endoscopic therapy for palliation of unresectable ampullary tumours.
iv. Comment on disorders predisposing to ampullary adenomas.
v. Comment on other malignant lesions of the papilla.

17 i. Squamous cell carcinoma of the anus; this is much less common than colorectal adenocarcinoma, but the distinction between the two is important because of therapeutic implications.
ii. Biopsy may sometimes be achieved endoscopically, but often needs to be performed with anaesthesia due to the very rich and sensitive cutaneous sensory nerve supply to this area.
iii. Human papilloma virus, condyloma acuminata and other venereal diseases, receptive anal intercourse in men, cigarette smoking and perianal Crohn's disease have been implicated as potential risk factors.
iv. Malignant neoplasms of the anal margin and canal metastasize to the superficial inguinal lymph nodes, while tumours proximal to the dentate line spread to the hypogastric nodes, along the inferior and middle haemorrhoidal vessels.
v. Treatment consists of radiotherapy and chemotherapy with 5-fluorouracil and mitomycin. In most cases, surgical intervention (i.e. abdominoperineal resection) is not needed for long-term survival.

18 i. It may be very difficult to confirm malignancy from endoscopic biopsies of the surface of a papillary tumour. It has been suggested that the yield of malignant tissue is increased by taking the biopsies from within an endoscopic papillotomy. Surgical resection and complete examination of the tissue obtained is the only way to determine the true nature of these tumours when endoscopic biopsies are benign.
ii. Ampullary cancer has a significantly better prognosis than ductal adenocarcinoma of the pancreas. It tends to grow locally without distant metastases. Enlarging papillary tumours may obstruct the duodenum, necessitating surgical gastric bypass.
iii. Endoscopic papillotomy and/or endoprosthesis (stent) placement palliates the jaundice and pruritus of ampullary tumours by relieving biliary obstruction. However, the risk of haemorrhage complicating endoscopic papillotomy is increased in the presence of a friable tumour, and the papillotomy site often occludes with further tumour growth. Endoscopic snare papillectomy has been used successfully to debulk papillary tumours, but there is a tendency for these to recur. This technique risks stenosis of the biliary and pancreatic duct orifices.
iv. In familial adenomatous polyposis (Gardner's syndrome), duodenal involvement frequently includes the duodenal papilla. Such patients require periodic screening endoscopy and biopsy of affected areas to look for dysplasia and malignancy.
v. Renal carcinoma has a particular predilection for the duodenal papilla when it metastasizes. Secondaries from malignant melanoma, and tumour deposits from other malignancies have also been found at this site.

19 A 10-year-old girl presented with a 3-month history of diarrhoea, abdominal pain and weight loss, taking her from the 50th to the 10th centile. She had been troubled by recurrent oral ulceration over the same period and had several times consulted her dentist. Topical steroids had ameliorated but not resolved the oral problem. In the week before presentation she had received a course of co-trimoxazole for a suspected urinary tract infection. On examination she was thin and there were several shallow ulcers of the buccal and sublingual mucosa. There was swelling of the lips, particularly the lower, with apparent thickening of the gums (19).

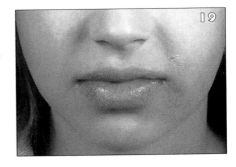

i. What is the differential diagnosis?
ii. What investigations are likely to be helpful?

20 A 30-year-old woman had a routine full blood count performed at a health screening medical which demonstrated an iron-deficiency anaemia with a haemoglobin of 9.6 g/dl, with normal white cell and platelet counts. Subsequent upper gastrointestinal endoscopy was macroscopically normal. Distal duodenal biopsies were taken (20a). A diagnosis was made and treatment initiated before further biopsy 3 months later (20b).

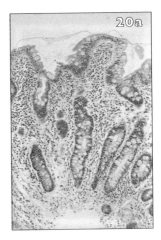

i. What abnormalities are seen in the two biopsies?
ii. What is the differential diagnosis?
iii. Which further investigations could be contributory?

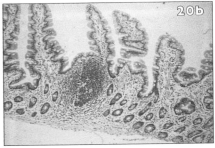

19 i. Crohn's disease is most likely given the gastrointestinal symptoms, but tuberculosis, Behçet's disease and coeliac disease may all present similarly. Orofacial granulomatosis, which she has (**19**), is most often linked to Crohn's disease when it is not idiopathic, but sarcoidosis is also a possibility and chest radiography is advisable. **ii.** The investigation most likely to provide diagnostic information in this patient is contrast radiology of the small bowel. This confirmed typical features of terminal ileal Crohn's disease and led to effective therapy with a combination of 1 month's exclusive defined formula nutritional therapy and subsequent maintenance with a slow-release mesalamine (mesalazine) preparation.

20 i. The first biopsy (**20a**) shows subtotal villous atrophy, crypt hyperplasia and a lymphocytic inflammatory infiltrate. There should not normally be more than one intra-epithelial lymphocyte for every three epithelial cells. **ii.** The appearances are typical of coeliac sprue, but other disorders which should be considered include tropical sprue, HIV-associated enteropathy, and Whipple's disease. The history is usually the most important guide to their relative likelihood. **iii.** Investigations which can be helpful include the estimation of red cell folate and barium examination of the small bowel. Only in the more severe symptomatic cases is it likely that other micronutrients will be deficient, but subclinical osteomalacia and impaired bone density is common in the untreated coeliac, warranting a check on vitamin D status. The biopsy can be studied immunohistochemically for the sub-type of lymphocyte in the inflammatory infiltrate. An increased proportion of intra-epithelial lymphocytes is characteristic of coeliac disease. Most patients with coeliac disease have serum antibodies to gliadin. Anti-endomysial antibody is more sensitive and very much more specific, with some authors even considering it a more reliable indicator than the presence of villous atrophy. Antibody diagnosis is, however, dependent on the ability of the patient to mount an IgA response.

21 This small-bowel barium study (21) was performed in a patient with altered bowel habit.
i. What abnormalities are shown?
ii. What is the diagnosis?
iii. Which is the gastrointestinal site most often implicated in this condition?
iv. What most characteristically happens in the colon when it is involved?

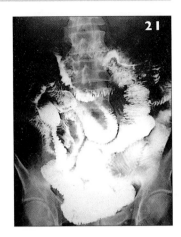

22 A 65-year-old woman with hypothyroidism and vitiligo complains of foul-smelling explosive diarrhoea preceded by abdominal cramping and bloating 1–2 hours after meals. There is a background of anaemia in the past for which she received a series of 'injections'. She discontinued this therapy a few years ago when she moved to another city. A blood profile now demonstrates a macrocytosis. A hydrogen breath test is included in the current work-up (22).
i. What underlying disorder does she have?
ii. How do you interpret the breath test results?
iii. How should she be treated?
iv. Should this patient be endoscoped?

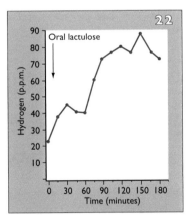

23 A 36-year-old man underwent upper gastrointestinal endoscopy for a 15-year history of epigastric pain.
i. What is the abnormality (23)?
ii. Is this likely to be the cause of the patient's symptoms?
iii. What are the associations of this condition?
iv. What is the treatment?

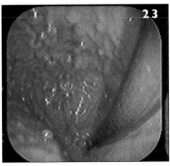

21 i. Marked dilatation of duodenum and jejunum with prominent, thickened valvulae conniventes (21).
ii. Intestinal scleroderma.
iii. The oesophagus (80% of those with GI disease).
iv. When the colon is affected there are typically wide-mouthed diverticula.

Gastrointestinal involvement occurs to a clinically relevant extent in about 50% of those with scleroderma. Oesophageal dysmotility is most common and may lead to serious nutritional deficit. Reflux coupled with poor oesophageal emptying, and associated oesophagitis frequently needs very high doses of proton pump inhibitors. Hypomotility of the small bowel, pseudo-obstruction, pneumatosis, generalized diverticulosis, intussusception, lymphangiectasia and volvulus are all seen. Malabsorption with steatorrhoea and small-bowel bacterial overgrowth are common.

22 i. This patient most likely has pernicious anaemia (PA) with small-bowel bacterial overgrowth from achlorhydria.
ii. 22 shows a high basal level which increases at 60 and 120 minutes after ingestion of lactulose. Normally, basal levels are low and increase when the ingested lactulose reaches the large bowel where it is digested by lactobacilli. Thus, the time to peak in a normal individual provides a measure of small-bowel transit. Here, this is the second peak whereas the first peak suggests bacterial overgrowth of the small bowel, leading to early lactulose digestion and early excretion of breath hydrogen. In the absence of a second peak, an early increase in breath hydrogen may signify a rapid small-bowel transit time or a shortened bowel (e.g. following resection), so clinical correlation is essential for correct interpretation.
iii. Therapy consists of intermittent antibiotics when symptoms warrant. Prophylactic maintenance antibiotics are generally not advised. Nutritional deficiencies must also be addressed.
iv. Although endoscopy may confirm the presence of gastritis and achlorhydria, a cancer surveillance role in established PA is controversial.

23 i. The number, sessile nature and fundal site suggest that these polyps are hyperplastic or regenerative. Gastric polyps are relatively rare: prevalence between 0.4 and 2%, of which 70% are hyperplastic. They are usually small and solitary. Diffuse hyperplastic polyposis as here (23) may represent a form of Ménétrier's disease. Histologically, these polyps consist of branching or elongated hyperplastic glands, often with a lymphocytic infiltrate. They are not true neoplasms and are without malignant potential.
ii. It is unlikely that these polyps are the cause of symptoms in the absence of bleeding or gastric outlet obstruction. Some 85% of those with gastric polyps have achlorhydria with a link to atrophic gastritis, pernicious anaemia and gastric carcinoma.
iii. Gastric polyposis occurs in familial adenomatous polyposis coli and in Peutz–Jegher's, Cowen's, and Cronkhite–Canada. True polyps are manifested rather than the hyperplastic lesions seen here.
iv. No treatment is necessary for these polyps, but adenomas are removed and regular endoscopic review conducted.

24 A 45-year-old man had surgery for a duodenal ulcer 15 years ago. For the past 4 years he has experienced intermittent diarrhoea.

i. Comment on the glucose/hydrogen breath test findings (24).
ii. What complications may ensue from this condition?
iii. What treatment may be indicated?

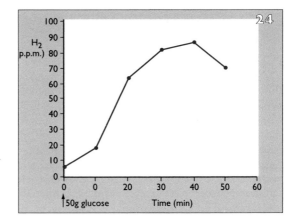

25 The colonoscopic appearances shown here (25) were noted in a 59-year-old woman with a long history of diarrhoea, for which no cause could be found.

i. What are these appearances?
ii. What is the cause and how might it be confirmed?
iii. What complications might this condition cause?

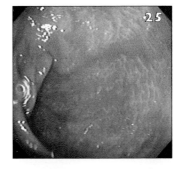

26 A 35-year-old housewife describes intermittent postprandial epigastric pain for 7 years. Cholecystectomy was ineffective. Endoscopy and ERCP proved normal. In the past she has had H2-receptor antagonists and cisapride, but with diminishing benefit. She denies weight loss, heartburn or alcohol intake but uses anti-inflammatory agents for menstrual pains. She is reluctant to undergo another endoscopic procedure but agrees to an upper GI series (26). A serum test for antibodies to *Helicobacter pylori* is positive.

i. What is this clinical entity?
ii. Discuss the differential diagnosis.
iii. Should any further testing be done?
iv. Should she be treated for *H. pylori* gastritis?

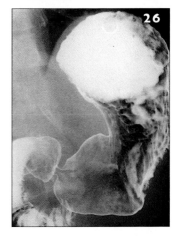

24 i. A rapid rise in breath hydrogen at 10 minutes (**24**) suggests small-bowel bacterial overgrowth. This occurs in 'blind loops' or other areas of stasis within the small bowel. The glucose/hydrogen breath test depends on the metabolism of glucose by bacteria, liberating hydrogen which can be measured in exhaled breath. An early sustained rise in breath hydrogen indicates overgrowth. The afferent loop of a Billroth II gastrectomy is an example of a 'blind loop'. Marked intraluminal proliferation of bacteria with a similar spectrum to that in the colon occurs and subsequent seeding of the whole small bowel can ensue.
ii. Generalized malabsorption may occur, leading to diarrhoea and malnutrition. Vitamin B_{12} is utilized by the proliferating bacteria and is unavailable for absorption. Deconjugation of bile salts in the proximal small intestine leads to failure of the enterohepatic circulation in the ileum, and subsequent fat malabsorption. Small-intestinal mucosal damage may occur, with enterocyte dysfunction, villous blunting and increased inflammatory infiltrate, further contributing to malabsorption.
iii. Treatment includes broad-spectrum antibiotics and corrective surgery. Treatment with antibiotics such as tetracyclines or ciprofloxacin is usually effective but bacterial overgrowth tends to return.

25 i. This is the typical 'tigroid' appearance of melanosis coli (**25**).
ii. It is caused by the chronic use of anthroquinone-containing laxatives, such as co-danthramer and senna. The microscopic appearances of macrophages laden with pigment (resembles lipofuscin) confirms the diagnosis. A history of laxative abuse is sought and can frequently be confirmed by screening the urine for metabolites of commonly used laxatives.
iii. Melanosis coli itself is, almost certainly, a benign condition, though some have suggested an association with colorectal carcinoma. Chronic laxative abuse may cause functional abnormalities of the myenteric plexus.

26 i. The primary cause here is dyspepsia. Although peptic ulcer is a common cause, the heterogeneous group of non-ulcer dyspepsias (NUDs) is more common still.
ii. NUD may be due to non-steroidal gastropathy, GORD, biliary tract disease, pancreatic disease, irritable bowel syndrome, gastric-emptying abnormality or non-gastrointestinal diseases.
iii. Because of the past surgery, post-cholecystectomy syndrome was considered and ERCP performed seeking retained bile duct stones. Bile may also be analysed for crystals, which predispose to recurrent pancreatitis. Sphincter of Oddi dysfunction, comfirmable by manometry, may lead to successful sphincterotomy, particularly if the bile duct is dilated and enzymes elevated. The primary therapeutic approach here is to discontinue NSAIDs.
iv. The role of antibiotic therapy directed against *H. pylori* gastritis in NUD remains controversial due to concerns regarding the potential for inducing antibiotic resistance, possible side effects of therapy and the absence of proved clinical benefit. Available data suggest that eradicating *H. pylori* fails to improve symptoms in most patients beyond the first few months after therapy. Antibiotic treatment may be offered with the understanding that its cost–benefit ratio is unknown.

27 A 26-year-old medical resident undertakes a short vacation in Acapulco, Mexico. He decides to 'immerse himself in regional culture' by sampling the local cuisine. Seventy-two hours after his arrival, he experiences the new onset of nausea, vomiting, flatulence, cramps, and copious watery diarrhoea. The hotel concièrge suggests that the medical resident is suffering from just another case of *turista* or travellers' diarrhoea, caused by a species of *Escherichia coli*. The resident prefers to describe his illness as 'Montezuma's revenge'.
i. Describe the spectrum of diseases caused by *E. coli*. Which species of *E. coli* is associated most commonly with travellers' diarrhoea?
ii. Which alarm symptoms would lead one to consider alternative diagnoses in the patient?
iii. Describe other pathogens which can cause diarrhoeal disease in travellers.
iv. Discuss the therapy of travellers' diarrhoea.
v. What is the role of prophylaxis?

28 A 27-year-old woman with a 1-year history of intermittent diarrhoea presents with itching.
i. Comment on the findings at ERCP (28).
ii. What is the diagnosis resulting in the presenting complaint?
iii. What other diagnosis may be present?
iv. What treatment options are available for the condition responsible for the itching?

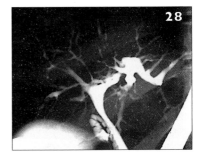

29 Mrs RC, a 34-year-old teacher, was diagnosed with ulcerative colitis approximately 8 years previously. She recently experienced a relapse which responded rapidly to a course of corticosteroid therapy. A barium enema is performed (29).
i. Comment on the radiological features.
ii. What options are available to decrease the propensity to relapse?
iii. Comment on any additional supplementation that may be necessary.
iv. Comment on maintenance therapy in Crohn's disease.

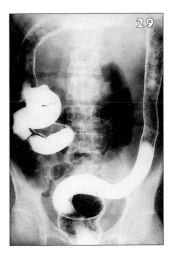

27 i. Five main categories of *E. coli* cause diarrhoea. Enteroinvasive *E. coli* is associated with outbreaks of mild-to-moderate disease. Enterohaemorrhagic *E. coli* is not truly invasive, but can cause severe haemorrhagic colitis and is associated with potentially lethal thrombotic thrombocytopenic purpura and haemolytic uraemic syndrome. Enterotoxigenic (ETEC), enteropathogenic, and enteroadherent *E. coli* cause diarrhoea by producing enterotoxins or by adhering to the intestinal brush border. ETEC causes diarrhoea in infants (primarily in developing nations), and is also the most common cause of travellers' diarrhoea. Less common non-invasive causes of travellers' diarrhoea include *Giardia lamblia* and *Cryptosporidium*.
ii. Severe systemic illness or rectal bleeding suggest invasive organisms as the cause.
iii. Invasive pathogens include: *Campylobacter*, *Salmonella*, *Shigella*, *Aeromonas*, *Plesiomonas*, *Entamoeba histolytica* and *Vibrio* species, other than *V. cholerae* which is a cause of toxigenic diarrhoea.
iv. Antibiotics are best avoided in patients with mild symptoms, as most diseases are self-limiting, but they reduce duration of symptoms in both children and adults. Antimotility agents (loperamide or diphenoxylate) may be used to control symptoms. Oral rehydration therapy is the first line of treatment in children.
v. This should be considered only for immunocompromised individuals.

28 i. The hepatic duct is dilated with a stricture in the left hepatic duct (**28**). The intrahepatic ducts are narrowed and shortened.
ii. Primary sclerosing cholangitis (PSC).
iii. Ulcerative colitis in >75% of patients, but much less often in Crohn's disease.
iv. Neither steroids nor azathioprine influence the course of the disease, which is apparently unaffected by colectomy. Indeed, PSC has been described presenting many years after panproctocolectomy. Selective stenting can be used when there is a dominant stricture in one of the major bile ducts. Ursodeoxycholic acid (ursodiol) has a choleretic effect and is apparently protective against damage to the biliary epithelium in animals. Human trials are not conclusive. Liver transplantation remains the only effective option once end-stage liver disease has supervened.

29 i. Tubular, ahaustral colon with granularity and occasional pseudopolyps of ulcerative colitis.
ii. Maintenance of remission in ulcerative colitis may be achieved with sulphasalazine, which is more effective than placebo and usually well tolerated. It is cheaper than mesalamine (mesalazine) preparations. Long-term immunosuppression may have unacceptable adverse effects, but is being utilized more frequently as a viable option for those with intractable symptoms, who cannot be weaned off corticosteroids, or in situations where deferral of proctocolectomy is desirable.
iii. Sulphasalazine is a competitive inhibitor of folic acid absorption; long-term use has been associated with folic acid deficiency. Folic acid 1 mg/day overcomes this problem.
iv. Maintenance of remission in Crohn's disease is more problematic. Mesalamine (mesalazine) and azathioprine are, however, effective in defined populations. The dose of 5-ASA needs to be higher than in ulcerative colitis. Maintenance therapy in Crohn's disease requires more individualization.

30 A businessman of Asian descent
presented with several months' general
malaise, right iliac fossa pain, and
intermittent diarrhoea. His job took
him all over the world, including
developing countries. On examination
there was tenderness in the right iliac
fossa and a low-grade fever.
Investigations revealed a mild
normocytic anaemia (haemoglobin
10.2 g/dl), an elevated CRP (55 mg/l),
and a sedimentation rate of 80 mm/h. A
radiological procedure was performed
(30).
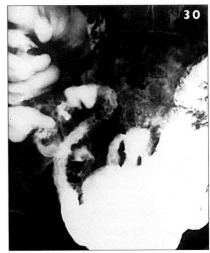
i. Describe what is seen.
ii. What is the differential diagnosis?
iii. How should he be further investigated?

31 A 25-year-old medical student is seen in the emergency room following a
celebration during which he consumed a large amount of alcohol. He began
to feel nauseated and then vomited up his dinner and some bilious material.
Shortly afterwards he vomited up about 150 ml of fresh blood. Apart from
some epigastric discomfort he did not volunteer any additional symptoms.
He was diagnosed with Christmas disease 10 years previously but had been
in excellent health until this episode. He did not smoke but admitted taking
alcohol over weekends to relieve the tensions of his work. He was found to
be comfortable with a pulse of 78/min and a blood pressure of
120/76 mmHg. The pulse rate increased to 104/min when he stood up, but
the blood pressure did not change significantly. Physical examination was
otherwise normal. The haemoglobin was 13.1 g/dl. An upper endoscopy
demonstrated a lesion at the oesophagogastric junction (31).
i. Comment on immediate emergency room
management.
ii. What is the likely diagnosis?
iii. Discuss confirmation of the diagnosis and
treatment of this patient.
iv. Comment on potential complications of the
gastrointestinal disorder and treatment this
particular patient may require.
v. Is the lesion likely to recur?

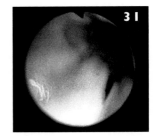

30 i. A barium follow through has been performed. There is (30) stricturing and ulceration of the terminal ileum. He has terminal ileitis.
ii. Crohn's disease, intestinal tuberculosis, yersiniosis, and lymphoma should be considered, although with an appropriate history, radiation damage might also be considered.
iii. Better imaging with a small-bowel enema might help, but a definitive diagnosis probably requires tissue for histological or microbiological assessment. Acute yersiniosis may however be confirmed by positive cultures of blood (or occasionally stool) and there are also fairly reliable serological tests. A chest radiograph is advised as this may help in the diagnosis of both tuberculosis and lymphoma, but the most productive investigation is ileoscopy at colonoscopy with biopsy. In this case the chest radiograph was normal, but characteristic caseating granulomas in the ileal biopsies which contained numerous acid-fast bacilli, made a diagnosis of intestinal tuberculosis straightforward. A final diagnosis is not always so easily reached. There was a good response to 9 months' antituberculous drug therapy. The chest radiograph is normal in approximately 50% of those presenting with intestinal tuberculosis in developed countries.

31 i. Intravenous access is obtained and intravascular volume maintained. Blood is taken for typing and cross-match. Infusion of an H2-receptor antagonist is beneficial (meta-analyses of outcome data) in upper gastrointestinal haemorrhage. The coagulation profile with a factor IX level is necessary to guide factor IX replacement. This patient is best managed in an intensive-care environment. A nasogastric tube is probably best avoided. Endoscopy is performed to establish a precise diagnosis and to treat any localized bleeding lesions.
ii. The history and circumstances support a clinical diagnosis of Mallory–Weiss tear – a linear laceration at the oesophagogastric junction – generally a feature of whatever caused the retching.
iii. The diagnosis is confirmed by endoscopy (31). The majority of lesions stop bleeding spontaneously and intervention is generally not required. Endoscopic haemostasis with electrocoagulation, or injection, stops the haemorrhage in most of those who continue to bleed, and surgery is rarely necessary. Purified factor IX concentrates may be necessary in Christmas disease (haemophilia B) and continued as for surgical levels of haemostasis (i.e. >30% at all times) until complete healing of the lesion.
iv. Surgery should be considered in intractable bleeding despite endoscopic intervention. Rarely, intramural haematomas may occur in patients with coagulopathy with minimal barotrauma. A very deep tear increases the risk of oesophageal rupture (Boerhaave's syndrome).
v. The endoscopy should have excluded other upper gastrointestinal pathology. He should be encouraged to discontinue alcohol which may predispose to further nausea and retching. Antisecretory agents are not protective, but the prognosis generally is excellent.

32 A 60-year-old man presents with complaints of nausea, vomiting, crampy abdominal pain and mild weight loss. There are no complaints of fever or night sweats. Physical examination reveals an element of muscle wasting and mild abdominal distention. Rectal examination is normal, but the stool is positive for occult blood. The haemoglobin is 11.2 g/dl with a borderline microcytosis. The barium enema is normal. A CT scan reveals focal thickening of the proximal small bowel wall, and luminal narrowing. A small-bowel follow-through radiograph is obtained (32a).

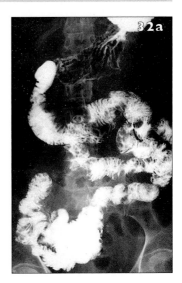

i. Describe the radiographic findings.
ii. What is the most likely diagnosis?
iii. How may the diagnosis be confirmed?
iv. What is the treatment for this condition?
v. Which complications may occur?

33 A 36-year-old male with regional enteritis for 17 years had multiple abdominal fistulae and short bowel syndrome. He was maintained on home parenteral nutrition, with oral intake contributing less than 10% of his diet. He was placed on antibiotics for control of his disease and recurrent urinary tract infections. He had previously been zinc deficient, which was corrected by adding extra zinc to the intravenous feed. He now presents with skin lesions around the eyes, nose and mouth (33) that were initially similar to those associated with his zinc deficiency, as well as hair loss. However, increasing his zinc supplementation to 12 mg/day i.v. does not correct the skin lesions, and the serum zinc level are in the normal range. The patient is receiving lipids with his intravenous feed, and does not have fatty acid deficiency.

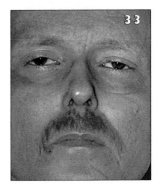

i. Discuss the differential for these skin lesions.
ii. What further assessment should be performed?
iii. What is the likely diagnosis?
iv. How else may this condition present?
v. What factors predisposed this patient to this problem?

32 i. A submucosal mass is present along the greater curvature, and marked nodularity is noted in the second, third, and fourth portions of the duodenum. More distally, multiple nodules protrude into the jejunum with multiple thickened folds.
ii. Lymphoma is the most common cause of nodular disease of the small bowel. Non-Hodgkin lymphoma accounts for 18–24% of all small-intestinal malignancies.

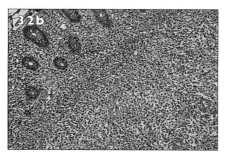

iii. Endoscopic biopsy of tissue of abnormal-appearance (32b) would assist. Bone marrow aspirate and biopsy, CT-guided fine needle biopsy of accessible masses, or laparoscopy are considered as alternatives to laparotomy (32c).

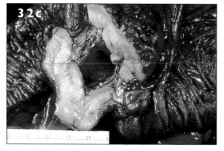

iv. Treatment of disseminated disease is with combination chemotherapy. Localized tumour masses, particular if painful, generally respond to radiotherapy. Most centres report 5-year survivals of around 50%. Surgical debulking has its advocates, but is not widely employed other than for isolated gastric lymphoma.
v. Bowel perforations may occur during therapy from rapid resolution of mural tumour, leaving a thin layer of tissue separating mucosa from peritoneum.

33 i. The differential diagnosis includes zinc deficiency, fatty acid deficiency, infectious causes such as *Candida*, and biotin deficiency.
ii. The lesions should be sampled for cytology and culture, and the plasma biotin level measured. A trial of intravenous biotin supplementation should rapidly improve the patient's skin lesions if there is biotin deficiency.
iii. Biotin deficiency. It is a cofactor for a number of carboxylases, but is abundant in food and also synthesized by intestinal flora. Dietary deficiency is therefore rare.
iv. It may present with scaly dermatitis (usually around the eyes, mouth and perineum); frequently there is hair loss and keratoconjunctivitis. Depression, lethargy, paraesthesia, muscle weakness and ataxia may also occur.
v. Abdominal fistulae increase biotin loss. Multiple antibiotics blocked bacterial production of biotin, and there was no biotin in his TPN solution.

34 A 6-month-old infant presents with a history of diarrhoea, poor weight gain and multiple infections including otitis media and cellulitis. Physical examination reveals clindactyly and an otitis media. Laboratory studies reveal a haemoglobin of 10.2 g/dl, WBC of 8.3×10^9/l (8300/mm^3) with only 700 neutrophils/mm^3. SGOT (AST), SGPT (ALT) and bilirubin are normal. The serum albumin is 29 g/l, and a small-bowel biopsy is normal.
i. What is the cause of the diarrhoea?
ii. Which disease entities may be responsible?
iii. What is the likely diagnosis?
iv. Describe the characteristics of this disorder.
v. What is the appropriate treatment?

35 A 36-year-old woman with familial hypertriglyceridaemia is hospitalized for recurrent pancreatitis. She denies any alcohol use or any medications associated with pancreatitis. She underwent a cholecystectomy following a prior episode of pancreatitis but no calculi were found to be present and her recurrent episodes continued. An ERCP performed after a prior episode 3 months previously was completely normal. The initial treatment consists of analgesia, intravenous maintenance solutions and nil by mouth. Her symptoms and initially elevated serum amylase and lipase settle after 5 days and a soft diet is introduced. However, she tolerates this poorly and her pain recurs, which is only partially relieved by vomiting. She is tender on examination and there is epigastric fullness with the suspicion of a mass. The serum amylase is now elevated again at 420 iu/l and lipase 610 u/l. The serum albumin is 22 g/l, haemoglobin 10.8 g/dl and WBC count 12.5×10^9/l (12 500/mm^3). The bilirubin is normal and ALP minimally elevated. There is no fever. A CT scan of the abdomen is performed (**35**).

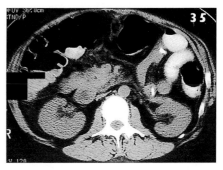

i. Why has the pain recurred?
ii. Comment on the features seen on the CT scan (**35**).
iii. Is an ERCP indicated?
iv. Comment on the serum albumin and what it may indicate.
v. Discuss management of this patient.

34 i. This presentation suggests malabsorption. The normal small-bowel and liver biochemistries make pancreatic disease the most likely cause.

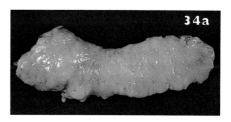

ii. Cystic fibrosis is the most common cause of pancreatic insufficiency in children. The severity of the dysfunction correlates with the type of *CFTR* gene mutation. Diagnosis requires a sweat chloride concentration of >60 mmol/l after stimulation by pilocarpine. DNA analysis is also helpful.

iii. The presence of neutropenia suggests the diagnosis of Schwachman syndrome.

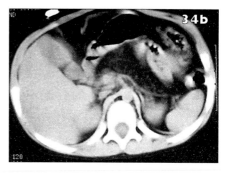

iv. It is characterized by short stature, exocrine pancreatic hypoplasia, a normal sweat chloride, cyclic neutropenia and skeletal changes. The pancreas is replaced by fat (**34a**), which can be demonstrated on abdominal CT (**34b**). Neutropenia may be intermittent. Thrombocytopenia and red cell hypoplasia may occur. Skeletal abnormalities include clindactyly, and rib and long-bone dysplasias.

v. Treatment consists of pancreatic enzyme replacement and treatment of associated infections.

35 i. Abdominal pain on re-feeding indicates that pancreatic inflammation has not resolved (despite overall improvement and resolution of the elevated serum amylase), probably as a result of stimulating pancreatic secretion.

ii. The CT demonstrates an enlarged pancreatic inflammatory mass with inflamed peritoneal fat – suggestive of pancreatic necrosis (phlegmonous pancreatitis). Abscess, pseudocyst and obstructed ductal system are not suggested.

iii. ERCP is not indicated. There is no evidence of an obstructed biliary system.

iv. This patient has on-going inflammatory disease (a catabolic state) and her current nutritional intake is suboptimal. Pancreatic rest (nil by mouth) is still required. Nutritional support is by the parenteral route. Placement of a nasoenteral tube beyond the ligament of Treitz, or laparoscopic-assisted placement of a jejunal tube, may be considered.

v. Pancreatic necrosis may take weeks to resolve, and domiciliary artificial nutrition is often appropriate. Oral enzymes or octreotide may be helpful, but remain untested. Antibiotics in the absence of infection are not helpful. Surgery is best resisted unless a complication (e.g. pancreatic abscess) intervenes. Hypertriglyceridaemia is treated. The reintroduction of oral feeds is determined clinically.

36 A 24-year-old, previously healthy graduate student returns from 2 months' travel in Eastern Europe with watery diarrhoea and cramping abdominal pain. Stool cultures reveal only normal flora. Flexible sigmoidoscopy is normal. His symptoms fail to respond to an empiric 5-day course of ciprofloxacin. Microscopy of the stool reveals the abnormality demonstrated in **36a** (arrow).

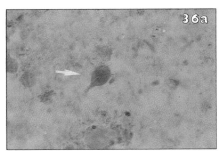

i. What is the most likely cause of the diarrhoea?
ii. How is the diagnosis generally confirmed?
iii. Describe the abnormality depicted in **36a** (arrow).
iv. Should any further diagnostic studies be performed?
v. How should the diarrhoea be treated?

37 A 23-year-old female college student presents with a history of nausea and vomiting and a 7 kg (15 lb) weight loss over the past 6 months. The patient does not believe that there is anything amiss, but describes only intermittent abdominal discomfort. She is accompanied by her parents who are quite concerned about her condition. The patient is a highly motivated, anxious, top-grade student who has not had health problems before, although the parents recall that she weighs herself frequently during home visits. The vomiting was first discovered by the parents. The patient developed facial swelling (**37**), which is the reason for her presentation. Her body weight is normal for her age and height. Physical examination demonstrates bilateral parotid enlargement but is otherwise unremarkable. Laboratory tests on initial evaluation were normal except for a serum amylase of 398 u/l (normal, <212 u/l).

i. What disease processes can be associated with asymptomatic parotid swelling such as that seen in (**37**)?

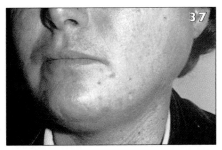

ii. What further laboratory tests are helpful in this patient?
iii. What is the probable diagnosis?
iv. What other gastrointestinal abnormalities may be seen in this condition?
v. Describe management of this patient.

36 & 37: Answers

36 i. *Giardia lamblia.* This protozoan particularly affects travellers to Eastern Europe and campers in the Rocky Mountains where the organism is present in the water supply. Human, dog, and beaver stools are the usual source.
ii. Diagnosis of giardiasis is difficult. At least three stool specimens are examined for cysts and active forms (**36a**). Sensitivity is improved by immunoprecipitation assay of the stool for *Giardia* antigens, but examination of a jejunal aspirate or proximal small-bowel biopsy (**36b**) may be needed as up to 50% of patients have no parasites in their stools.

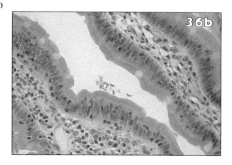

iii. The stool examination reveals active forms of *Giardia lamblia.*
iv. Once confirmed, no further testing is necessary.
v. Giardiasis responds to metronidazole, quinacrine or furazolidone, which may be employed empirically if the diagnosis is strongly suspected.

37 i. Alcoholic cirrhosis, nutritional deficiencies and malabsorption, Sjögren's syndrome, drugs, uraemia, amyloidosis, mumps, infectious mononucleosis, Lyme disease, recurrent vomiting and eating disorders (bulimia nervosa) may all be associated. Solid tumours are seldom bilateral.
ii. The amylase could be of salivary or pancreatic origin. A serum isoamylase or a serum lipase is helpful. CT or ultrasound of the pancreas may help, but abnormalities can also be seen in eating disorders. A nutritional analysis and tests for connective tissue disorders are useful. The serum lipase proved normal, and the isoamylase showed an elevated salivary fraction, confirming its salivary origin.
iii. Bulimia nervosa. The young age, female sex and compulsive nature fit well. Furthermore, the parents initially discovered the secretive vomiting, and parotid enlargement is associated with self-induced vomiting. Calluses or scarring may be found on the back of the hand used to induce vomiting (Russell's sign).
iv. Eating disorders are associated with delayed gastric emptying and delayed small-bowel transit. Rectal impaction may occur in patients with poor oral intake. Rarely, there may be re-feeding pancreatitis or problems from inspissated secretions in the pancreatic duct. Dental abnormalities include loss of dental enamel, and cavities from chronic vomiting.
v. Patients with suspected eating disorders need psychiatric evaluation and a multidisciplinary approach. Abdominal complaints are not unusual and 25% of patients have electrolyte abnormalities. Adequate hydration is particularly important for those with parotid enlargement. Salivary secretions contribute importantly to oesophageal mucosal integrity and their absence predisposes to distal oesophagitis.

38 A 43-year-old nurse's aide is transferred from another hospital with a 6-month history of high-volume watery diarrhoea. She has been hospitalized four times with dehydration and hypokalaemia. An extensive evaluation including barium contrast studies and secretory hormones was unrevealing. Laboratory results include potassium 2.9 mmol/l and magnesium 0.9 mmol/l. A flexible sigmoidoscopy demonstrates an abnormal mucosal pattern (38).

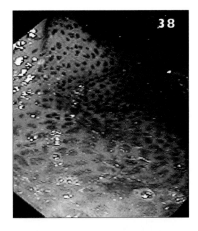

i. Describe the endoscopic appearances.
ii. What type of diarrhoea does the patient have?
iii. How may the diagnosis be confirmed?
iv. Comment on the patient profile commonly seen with this disorder.
v. How is this disorder treated?

39 A 40-year-old woman presents for investigation of recurrent episodes of pancreatitis dating back at least 5 years. A prior ERCP attempt failed to demonstrate the pancreatic duct. Repeat ERCP (39a, 39b) through the main duodenal papilla reveals an unusually short pancreatic duct.

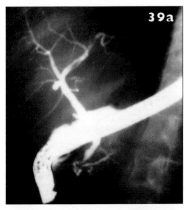

i. Which additional blood tests may prove useful in evaluating the aetiology of recurrent pancreatitis?
ii. Describe the ERCP abnormality present in 39a.
iii. Describe the structure identified in 39b.
iv. How do these appearances relate to the patient's relapsing pancreatitis?
v. Is endoscopic therapy indicated, and if so, what type?

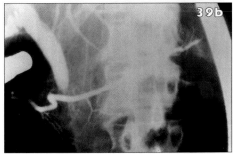

38 i. Characteristic pigmentation of melanosis coli from chronic anthraquinone laxative use.
ii. Factitious diarrhoea due to surreptitious laxative use which is secretory in nature and with a reduced stool osmotic gap.
iii. Melanosis is not a reliable sign, and the diagnosis must be confirmed by a stool laxative screen or a room search.
iv. Melanosis is most frequently seen in middle-aged and elderly women. Many patients are paramedical. The other subset of those with factitious diarrhoea is younger women with atypical eating disorders.
v. Gentle confrontation and psychiatric consultation are appropriate but are frequently rebuffed by patients, who tend to deny laxative use and seek medical attention elsewhere. Those that accept the diagnosis often develop constipation and considerable abdominal discomfort when the laxatives are withdrawn, and constitute a considerable management challenge. Neurological damage to the colon may occur, resulting in an atonic, functionless organ.

39 i. Those for hypertriglyceridaemia, hypercalcaemia, autoimmune disease, cystic fibrosis, renal disease, drugs, infective agents and granulomatous disorders. A blood alcohol screen proves useful if abuse is suspected.
ii. A small ventral pancreatic ductal system has been opacified. This may be differentiated from an abrupt blockage (e.g. malignant stricture) by the fine terminal arborization of the duct. It usually suggests pancreas divisum. This variant, present in 7–8% of Caucasian patients, results when the two embryonic buds (**39c**, item a) of the foregut that form the pancreas fail to fuse after rotation, leaving separate ductal systems (**39c**, item b). The larger, dorsal pancreatic duct (D) empties into the duodenum via the accessory (minor) papilla. The smaller ventral duct (V) empties via the main (major) duodenal papilla. (**39c**, item c is the normal fused ductal system.)
iii. A normal-appearing dorsal pancreatic duct has been opacified.
iv. The relationship of pancreas divisum to recurrent pancreatitis and chronic pancreatic pain is controversial. Although pancreas divisum may be an incidental finding, mechanical obstruction to exocrine secretion from the dorsal duct, either from stenosis or sphincter dysfunction, may occur and cause pancreatitis.
v. There are limited data regarding the use of endoscopic therapy in pancreas divisum. The best results of minor sphincterotomy are seen in pancreas divisum patients with recurrent discrete episodes of pancreatitis (70% cure rate). The least successful sphincterotomies are in those with continuous pain – the results equate to placebo.

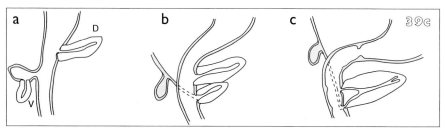

40 A 36-year-old man presents with a 2-year history of rectal bleeding. There is no weight loss nor family history of colon cancer. Colonoscopy is performed. The findings seen in (40a) are found throughout the colon and rectum. Histological examination of three of these lesions reveals tubular adenomas.

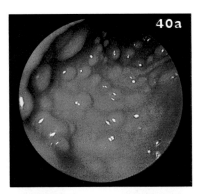

i. Describe the lesions shown.
ii. Comment on the genetics of this disorder.
iii. How should family members be managed?
iv. What is the risk of colorectal carcinoma in this patient?
v. Comment on extracolonic manifestations of this disease.

41 A 72-year-old man is hospitalized in the intensive care unit for treatment of Gram-negative sepsis secondary to a urinary tract infection. Treatment includes low-dose dopamine in view of hypotension. After 24 hours, the patient develops excruciating abdominal pain. Physical examination reveals minimal abdominal tenderness that is non-focal. There is no stool in the rectal vault and mucus is negative for occult blood. An emergency angiogram (41a) demonstrates attenuated mesenteric arteries. A normal angiogram (41b) is shown for comparison.

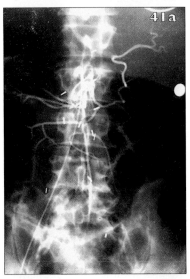

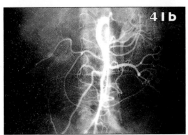

i. What is the diagnosis?
ii. Discuss the pathogenesis of this condition.
iii. How should the diagnosis be confirmed?
iv. What treatment options are available?
v. What other conditions enter into the differential diagnosis?

40 i. Profuse polyposis of familial adenomatous polyposis (FAP).
ii. This arises from mutation of the *APC* gene on chromosome 5, and is inherited as an autosomal dominant. 'Sporadic' new mutations account for 33% of cases.
iii. Sporadic cases pose the same risk to future generations, so children of probands must be screened (every 1–2 years from

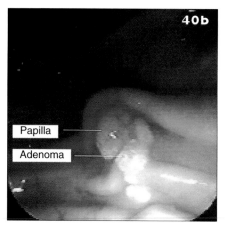

10–12 years). Polyps are first detectable at a mean age of 16 years, but cause symptoms much later (mean of 36 years). **iv.** The risk of colorectal cancer approaches 95% by the age of 50, so proctocolectomy is advised. **v.** Most FAP patients develop duodenal adenomas, mainly of the periampullary area (**40b**). The lifetime risk of duodenal cancer is 5–10%, so duodenoscopy every 1–3 years is wise. Fundic gland polyps are commonly present and are not premalignant. Desmoid tumours cause considerable morbidity in FAP patients and result in death in up to 10%.

41 i. Non-occlusive mesenteric ischaemia.
ii. Acute occlusive mesenteric ischaemia is usually caused by an embolus to the superior mesenteric artery. Non-occlusive ischaemia occurs in settings of 'low-flow', and is associated with hypotension. Both may cause infarction of the bowel. Abdominal pain is the norm, but distension and ileus may be the presenting features in unconscious patients hospitalized with critical illness.
iii. Tissue necrosis may lead to fever, leukocytosis, rebound tenderness, abdominal distension, or lactic acidosis. Survival is dependent on early diagnosis. Mesenteric angiography may not be necessary before laparotomy if the diagnosis is strongly suspected. CT may confirm the diagnosis and exclude other causes of ileus in a shocked patient. Undue surgical delay, however, may compromise potentially salvageable bowel.
iv. The patient's haemodynamic condition must be stabilized with fluid resuscitation and discontinuation of vasoconstricting drugs. Intra-arterial infusion of papaverine, a vasodilating drug, or a thrombolytic may be helpful. Laparotomy may permit embolectomy and is required to resect necrosed bowel. Unfortunately, mortality is high and many of those who survive are left with a shortened bowel.
v. Most patients have abdominal tenderness. Although mesenteric ischaemia often presents with pain out of proportion to the physical signs, pancreatitis, ruptured or dissecting aortic aneurysm, perforated abdominal viscus and strangulated abdominal viscera may need to be considered.

42 A 5-year-old boy presented with a 12-month history of upper abdominal pain, and a longer past history of recurrent mouth ulcers. There had been a slight drop in his growth centiles, and his parents and teacher described him as increasingly moody. There were no other symptoms. On examination, no ulcers were seen, but he looked miserable and there was possibly some abdominal distension. Initial investigations were as in the table.
i. What is the most likely diagnosis and why?
ii. What investigations are best suited to confirm the diagnosis?

Investigation	Result
Haemoglobin	8.2 g/dl
MCV	101 fl
MCH	28 pg
White cell count	8.0 × 10⁹/l with normal differential
Urea and electrolytes	Normal
Albumin	24 g/l
ESR	15 mm/h
CRP	1 mg/l
IgA	0.3 g/l (normal 0.9–4.5 g/l)
IgG	9 g/l (normal 8–18 g/l)
IgM	1.2 g/l (normal 0.8–2.4 g/l)

43 A 28-year-old woman presents to the emergency room with severe central abdominal pain which is constant, but with a colicky component. Her history is remarkable for episodic attacks of abdominal discomfort, less severe than the current episode, that may last for many hours. She has vomited on occasion and felt slightly distended. Although she is constipated during these attacks, a tendency to loose stools lasts for a few days afterwards. She also reports swelling of her arms, legs and lips with minimal trauma. The swelling is non-tender, and unaccompanied by rash or pruritus. She has experienced occasional respiratory difficulty which has been attributed to an allergic diathesis. She denies any fever or rashes and is otherwise in excellent health. Her mother experienced similar problems but died of asphyxia after a surgical procedure. Examination demonstrates mid-abdominal tenderness with no distention or peritonism. Bowel sounds are high-pitched. The blood and differential counts are within normal limits. Barium radiography was performed (43).
i. Describe the radiological abnormality.
ii. Discuss the differential diagnosis.
iii. What further investigations are useful?
iv. Discuss the pathophysiology of this disorder.
v. Comment on treatment of this disorder.

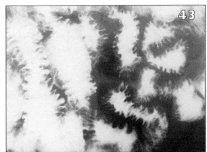

42 i. This is coeliac disease.
ii. The combination of folate deficiency with IgA deficiency is typical of coeliac disease, although iron deficiency is also frequently seen. The folate may fall again rapidly after initial correction on introduction of a gluten-free diet, making folate particularly helpful in monitoring progress. IgA endomysial antibody and antigliadin antibodies are found in both children and adults with untreated coeliac disease. A low total IgA may, however, mask this phenomenon and probably accounts for most of the false-negative antibody tests. Some children truly lack endomysial antibodies, and very occasionally they are detected in other enteropathies. The relevant tests, therefore, are antiendomysial antibodies and small-bowel biopsy, the latter normally showing characteristic villous atrophy and excess intraepithelial lymphocytes.

43 i. The barium study demonstrates diffuse thickening of small-bowel folds. No stenoses, ulceration or masses are apparent.
ii. This suggests thickening of the small-bowel wall by blood (as in coagulopathy or following trauma), oedema, cellular infiltration (mastocytosis, eosinophilia, amyloid, granulomatous disease) or extensive tumour infiltration.
iii. The history suggests angio-oedema which may be primary, or secondary to a systemic disorder. There is little to suggest an allergic disorder or malignancy, and the family history suggests the hereditary form. This is characterized by low functional levels of C1 inhibitor activity and, as a result of failure of the C1 inhibitor to block the enzymatic activity of C1. Levels of C4 and C2 are reduced. There is an association with autoimmune disorders, and SLE should be excluded. In view of the radiology it is also appropriate to exclude disordered coagulation.
iv. Hereditary angio-oedema is an autosomal dominant disorder characterized by deficiency of a complement cascade regulatory protein, C1 esterase inhibitor. C1 inhibits C1r and C1s in the complement system, Factor XII and kallikrein in the contact system, and Factor XI in the coagulation system. Histamine plays no role. The C1 inhibitor gene is on chromosome 11p and variants are due to small mutations, deletions and insertions. In type I disease, the protein product is absent or low, whereas in type II disease, present in 15% of affected patients, there is a dysfunctional protein; these patients have normal or elevated levels of C1 inhibitor antigen – but the functional assay is abnormal. The disease is characterized by bouts of non-pitting oedema of the extremities, larynx, face and abdomen. Without treatment, mortality from upper airway obstruction may exceed 25%.
v. Replacement therapy with C1 inhibitor concentrates is used for laryngeal oedema and severe abdominal attacks. Vapour-heated C1 inhibitor concentrate is preferred, being of lower viral risk than that derived from plasma. Androgens increase the synthesis of C1 and can be used to prevent attacks triggered by oropharyngeal (dental) manipulations, but must be given for 5 days beforehand (and not in pregnant and prepubertal patients). Simple subcutaneous swelling is best left untreated.

44 A young woman presented with increasing dysphagia. She had noticed that she could no longer eat as fast as other members of her family, but denied weight loss. Her partner had commented on her bad breath. Examination was unremarkable. There were no neurological signs or lymphadenopathy. Following investigation she agreed to therapeutic endoscopy (44).
i. What is the differential diagnosis?
ii. What has happened?
iii. Describe the physical signs to be expected.
iv. Describe the next steps in management.

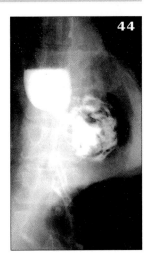

45 A 32-year-old motor cyclist was admitted after a road traffic accident with a transection of his cervical spinal cord at C8 and an almost total quadriplegia. His condition was complicated by septicaemia attributed to infection of a central venous feeding line. Treatment with high-dose floxacillin (flucloxacillin), ampicillin and gentamicin was commenced, with initial improvement. He was noted to be constipated until day 12 at which point voluminous diarrhoea began. At the same time he described dysphagia for solids and liquids. His initial fever then recurred and his white blood cell count again rose. There were no new physical signs otherwise. Upper GI endoscopy (45a) and sigmoidoscopy (45b) were performed.

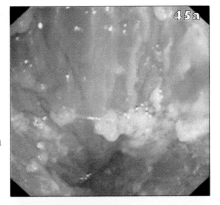

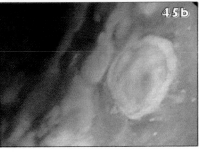

i. Describe the appearances and outline the likely explanations.
ii. Could these problems have been prevented?
iii. How does the neurological defect impact on the GI management?

44 & 45: Answers

44 i. The differential diagnosis includes functional disorders, achalasia and neoplasia. Investigation included barium swallow which showed the typical 'rat's tail' appearance of achalasia.
ii. Oesophageal manometry confirmed the raised resting pressure of the lower oesophageal sphincter and a failure of its relaxation with swallowing. Endoscopically guided balloon disruption of the lower oesophageal sphincter was the chosen therapy, but unfortunately this was complicated by perforation as demonstrated on the water-soluble contrast swallow examination.
iii. There may be pain and distress but the classic sign is of surgical emphysema in the upper chest and neck progressing to features of septicaemic shock if the problem is not recognized and acted upon.
iv. Management should have commenced before the procedure, as this is a recognized complication and should have figured in the explanation to the patient when obtaining informed consent. If there is suspicion of perforation (from endoscopic appearances or early symptoms or signs), a water-soluble contrast study is performed. Barium should not be used, as serious mediastinitis occurs if there is a perforation. A nil-by-mouth regime, with broad-spectrum antibiotics and parenteral feeding, sometimes suffices, but surgical advice is always sought at the earliest opportunity as the timing of surgical intervention needs to be carefully chosen for best results.

45 i. **45a** shows oesophageal candidiasis and **45b** shows pseudomembranous colitis, characterized by white plaques adherent to an erythematous mucosa and yellowish plaques on a grey-coated mucosa.
ii. It would be unusual for a previously fit individual to develop oesophageal candidiasis after a short course of broad-spectrum antibiotics. Additional predisposing factors are accordingly sought. Pseudomembranous colitis, however, is adequately explained by antibiotic use. Fluconazole and metronidazole given orally should normally suffice.
iii. Afferent sensory input from the oesophagus travels mainly by the sympathetics to the spinal cord between C1 and L3. These nerves also supply efferent fibres to the oesophagus from T4 to L2. Motor function is otherwise either from spinal roots above C8 or vagal, and is unaffected in a case such as this. The absence of afferent fibres may explain why the candidiasis was unassociated with pain. The dysphagia was considered to be of infective origin with no neurological component.

After major spinal injury there is usually slow-transit constipation and disordered defaecation, sometimes with reflex defaecation as the rectum fills. It is probable that the diarrhoea in this case was a result of the colitis. Impaired gastric emptying is common in spinal injury, often with gastro-oesophageal reflux. In autonomic dysreflexia, injury proximal to the splanchnic outflow at T5 is responsible for faecal impaction together with profound hypertension and tachycardia. This can prove fatal if not recognized and treated promptly with laxatives, and is better prevented by their routine use from the time of admission.

46 Shown (46) is the oesophagus of a
54-year-old publican/bartender.
i. Describe the findings at endoscopy
(46).
ii. What is the most likely aetiology?
iii. List the therapeutic options in the
event of an acute bleed.

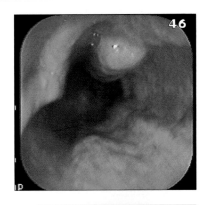

47 A 55-year-old man presents with fatigue
and intermittent black stools. He has
experienced occasional periumbilical
cramping, particularly a few hours after
eating. He has lost 2.2 kg (5 lb) in weight over
the previous 3 months. His past history is
remarkable for indigestion for which he uses
regular antacids, and an old knee injury for
which he takes ibuprofen on an as-needed
basis. Physical examination reveals pallor, but
is otherwise unremarkable. Occult blood is
positive in the stool. Haemoglobin is 8.8 g/dl,
MCV is 72 fl. Upper

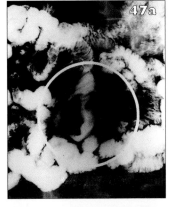

endoscopy reveals a number of
pre-pyloric erosions. A
colonoscopy is normal.
i. Discuss the differential
diagnosis.
ii. Discuss additional testing
that may be indicated.
iii. Comment on the
abnormalities detected by the
radiological examinations in
47a and 47b.
iv. Comment on the diagnostic
possibilities at this stage.
v. Discuss management of the patient.

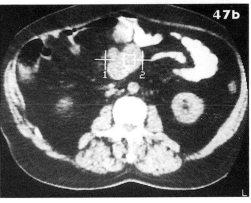

46 & 47: Answers

46 i. There are four cords of oesophageal varices (**46**). There are no signs indicative of impending or recent haemorrhage.

ii. Alcoholic cirrhosis is most likely, but any cause of portal hypertension results in varices. The differential diagnosis is therefore wide.

iii. Following the initial resuscitation the patient is endoscoped promptly; treatment options include:
- Injection sclerotherapy using a sclerosant, an adhesive, or bovine thrombin. Sclerotherapy may be repeated in the event of a rebleed.
- Banding using a multiple ligation device; it is probable that banding is safer than sclerotherapy and possible that it is more efficacious.

Other measures include:
- Balloon tamponade, a useful holding measure in the event of uncontrolled haemorrhage.
- Drugs – vasopressin, glypressin or octreotide are all of value in selected patients.
- Surgery – oesophageal transection, portosystemic shunts (surgical or TIPSS).

47 i. Melaena, food-related abdominal pain, NSAID use and a background of dyspepsia suggest a gastroduodenal origin. However, the endoscopy fails to demonstrate a convincing cause. The colonoscopy excludes a source in the colon. Mesenteric ischaemia is a cause of postprandial pain, but there are no other risk factors for vascular disease. Arteriovenous malformations in the small bowel, and Meckel's diverticulum cause blood loss, but not weight loss. The pain may indicate clot-induced colic or luminal stenosis. Crohn's disease rarely presents with bleeding. Neoplasia needs to be excluded. Gastric erosions are an insufficient explanation.

ii. Additional investigations include small-bowel barium study, enteroscopy, and CT if a mass lesion is found. Scintigraphy is generally unhelpful in the absence of on-going active bleeding. Mesenteric arteriography is, however, sometimes useful.

iii. The follow-through demonstrates a constricting ileal lesion producing an 'apple-core' appearance. The CT scan demonstrates a mass in this area.

iv. These suggest a neoplasm, probably adenocarcinoma – which represents 50% of small-bowel tumours. Carcinoid tumours account for about 30%, lymphomas 15% and leiomyosarcomas about 10–13% of small-bowel malignant lesions in most series. A benign cause is unlikely on radiological grounds.

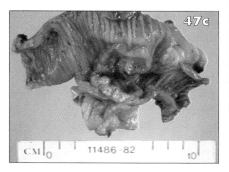

v. With high suspicion of cancer, and low-grade obstructive symptoms, laparotomy with resection of the stenotic lesion is indicated (**47c**). A CT-guided biopsy of the mass would be reasonable preoperatively, but is unlikely to alter a decision to proceed with surgery. Similarly, enteroscopy has little to offer.

48 A 22-year-old man has had
abdominal bloating and diarrhoea
for 3 months. A duodenal biopsy
(48) is performed after a series of
normal laboratory investigations.
i. What does the biopsy show?
ii. What factors in the history should
have been sought?
iii. What, if any, further
investigations are appropriate?

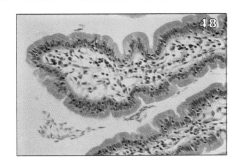

49 A male patient has had extensive ulcerative colitis for 4 years, quiescent
on sulphasalazine. For 2 months he has experienced pruritus, fatigue, and
darkening of the urine. Examination is unremarkable. A blood count is
within normal limits but the bilirubin is
60 μmol/l (3.5 mg/dl) and ALP is 295 u/l (normal
<110 u/l). Ultrasound examination was normal.
An ERCP is performed (49).
i. What is the differential diagnosis?
ii. What pathological findings are expected on
liver biopsy?
iii. With which disease is the presenting disorder
most commonly associated?
iv. Does bowel resection influence the natural
history of this disease?
v. Comment on other hepatobiliary
manifestations of inflammatory bowel disease.

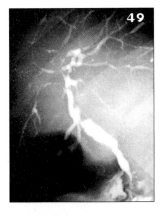

50 Shown (50) is the barium study of a 50-year-
old woman who presented with abdominal pain,
diarrhoea and occasional vomiting. There was a
past history of ovarian cancer.
i. What are the radiological abnormalities and
what is the likely diagnosis?
ii. Does surgery have any role?

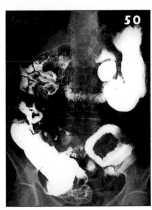

48–50: Answers

48 i. *Giardia lamblia* parasites are present in the small-bowel lumen; the villous architecture is preserved (**48**).
ii. Other aspects of the history of possible relevance therefore include foreign travel, or evidence of immunodeficiency.
iii. This infection has a world-wide distribution but is more common in under-developed countries. Symptoms may be absent or result in diarrhoea, bloating and pain. The stools are frequently very loose and watery with steatorrhoea. Both cysts and trophozoite forms may be present in the stools, but in 50% of infections neither is detectable. Examination of duodenal aspirates, and biopsies are more sensitive. Eosinophilia is not associated. Deficiency of IgA and more generalized immunodeficiency (as in HIV infection) accounts for most cases that prove resistant to simple therapy with metronidazole or tinidazole.

49 i. Primary sclerosing cholangitis (PSC) may be confirmed by cholangiography in the absence of secondary sclerosing cholangitis (prior biliary surgery, choledocholithiasis). Typical features include intrahepatic ductal narrowing and extrahepatic ductal stenosis. Prestenotic ductal dilatation also can be seen (**49**).
ii. Liver biopsy exhibits extrahepatic cholestasis with neutrophils in the portal tract and, later, secondary biliary cirrhosis with 'onion skinning' of the portal tract.
iii. Sclerosing cholangitis is more common in males and is seen in at least 2% of those with ulcerative colitis but in less than 1% of those with Crohn's disease.
iv. Treatment of the bowel does not influence the liver disease. There is no known useful therapy for PSC, although ursodiol (ursodeoxycholic acid) often improves the pruritus and decreases enzyme elevation. When cirrhosis with decompensation intervenes, orthotopic liver transplantation is a viable option.
v. Other hepatobiliary manifestations of inflammatory bowel disease include cholelithiasis, steatosis, amyloidosis, and cholangiocarcinoma.

50 i. There are multiple small-bowel strictures, dilatation and mucosal irregularities suggestive of ulceration (**50**). It is probable that this represents radiation enteritis.
ii. Surgery has a limited role in therapy because of the high risk of anastomotic breakdown and enterocutaneous fistulae and is reserved for complete obstruction, major haemorrhage, perforation or secondary malignancy. Up to 15% of patients in whom the small intestine is inevitably in the radiation field develop radiation enteritis. It is less often seen with better radiotherapy planning, but still occurs unpredictably with correctly planned radiation exposure that causes no problems in others. In the acute phase there is villous shortening and thinning of the mucosa, associated with diarrhoea and, sometimes, with bleeding. This usually resolves completely. Sub-acute disease with progressive vascular damage and ischaemic fibrosis occurs 2–12 months after exposure, and may go on to chronic disease where mucosal and submucosal changes extend to the muscularis and serosa. This may be progressive and many patients present as late as 10 years after exposure but then follow a chronic progressive course. Management is predominantly supportive and may require intravenous nutrition on a long-term basis.

51 A 5-week-old baby has the gradual onset of non-bilious projectile vomiting, scleral icterus and decreased urine output. He was breast-fed until 3 weeks of age and then changed to a cows' milk-based formula. Physical examination reveals a lethargic infant with a sunken anterior fontanelle and dry mucous membranes. He does not produce tears when crying. His abdomen distends until he forcefully vomits, when distention resolves. A 2×3 cm mobile mass is palpable in the epigastric region. Laboratory blood tests reveal: sodium 135 mmol/l, potassium 2.8 mmol/l, chloride 88 mmol/l, bicarbonate 32 mmol/l, SGOT (AST) 34 u/l, SGPT (ALT) 28 u/l, total bilirubin 119 μmol/l (7 mg/dl), conjugated bilirubin 13.6 μmol/l (0.8 mg/dl).
i. What is the most probable diagnosis?
ii. Describe the classic clinical sign of this entity.
iii. How may the diagnosis be confirmed?
iv. Explain the metabolic abnormalities and hyperbilirubinaemia.
v. What is the management of this patient?

52 A 12-month-old child presented with failure to thrive. He was born at 33 weeks' gestation with a birthweight of 2.1 kg (4.7 lb) (50th centile), and was nursed in neonatal intensive care but did not require ventilation. Initially, he was fed with pre-term formula and subsequently bottle-fed well. At 4 weeks he weighed 2.9 kg (6.4 lb) (50th centile), and was discharged home well. He followed the 50th centile until 5 months. At 5 months he started to wake screaming and, although he could be consoled by feeding, he often woke again after a few hours. Vomiting started at 8 months and by this time his growth had slowed to the 10th centile. The table below and 52 show the results of gastro-oesophageal pH studies.
i. What is the diagnosis?
ii. What is the management in this situation?

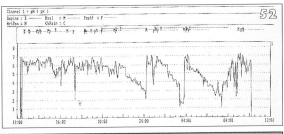

Acid Reflux		Total	Upright	Supine	Meal	PostP
Duration	(h:min)	21:46	11:16	10:30	03:40	13:46
Number of reflux episodes		154	21	134	2	40
Number of reflux episodes longer than 5.0 minutes		7	0	7	0	2
Longest reflux episode	(min)	45	2	45	1	9
Total time pH below 4.00	(min)	173	6	157	3	29
Fraction time pH below 4.00	(%)	13.3	0.9	25.6	1.2	3.5

51 & 52: Answers

51 i. Idiopathic hypertrophic pyloric stenosis.
ii. A mobile pyloric mass, similar in size and shape to an olive in the epigastrium.
iii. Ultrasonography reveals a thickened (>3 mm), elongated pyloric muscle wall
(51a). Alternatively, gastrointestinal contrast study reveals characteristic elongation
and narrowing of the pyloric canal (51b). Endoscopy is usually not required (51c).

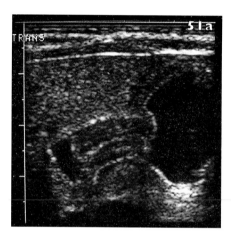

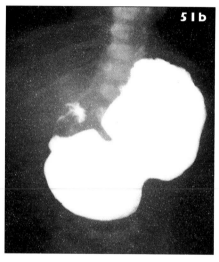

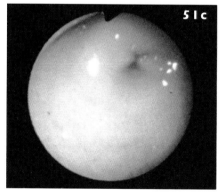

iv. Prolonged vomiting leads to
dehydration and hypochloraemic
alkalosis. Unconjugated
hyperbilirubinaemia (in about 5% of
cases) is thought to be due to inadequate
absorption of glucose and an inability to
maintain glucuronyl transferase activity.
v. Resuscitation and then a Ramstedt
pyloromyotomy.

52 i. Gastro-oesophageal reflux.
ii. Frequent small feeds usually help. Continuous nasogastric tube drip feeding is
effective in more severe cases and may help to avoid surgical intervention so long as
catch-up growth begins within 7 days. Thickening the feeds is also helpful. Acid-
reducing agents help if oesophagitis has occurred. Promotility agents increase resting
lower oesophageal sphincter pressure and increase anterograde gastric emptying;
cisapride is probably most effective and least likely to cause side effects.

53 Match each of the following cells (i–v) with the appropriate function
(a–e) regarding gastric acid secretion.
i. Enterochromaffin-like cell (ECL cell).
ii. Antral G-cell.
iii. Antral D-cell.
iv. Parietal cell.
v. Mucus neck cell.
a. Possesses gastrin receptors, muscarinic receptors and histamine receptors
which, when bound, stimulate it to produce its secretory product.
b. Its main role is inhibitory control of gastric acid secretion.
c. Secretes bicarbonate and water as well as other products.
d. Secretes gastrin in response to gastric luminal nutrients and gastrin-
releasing peptide (GRP), and is inhibited in the presence of acid.
e. Releases histamine in response to gastrin binding to its
gastrin/cholecystokinin (CCK)-B receptor.

54 A 28-year-old labourer, a recent immigrant from South America, has lower
abdominal cramping pain of 4 weeks' duration, bloody diarrhoea and weight
loss. He was unresponsive to antidiarrhoeals and a 1-week course of a
sulphonamide. He has managed to continue to work with difficulty due to
progressive fatigue. He is heterosexual and does not smoke or consume
excessive alcohol. Examination reveals him to be slightly pale with a
temperature of 37°C (98.5°F) and a heart rate of 94/min. The cardiovascular
and respiratory systems are unremarkable. There is
mild muscle wasting, and a non-distended abdomen
with generalized tenderness, worse on the left side, but
no peritonism. Bowel sounds are normal. Stools are
overtly bloody. Stool culture is negative. Colonoscopy
demonstrates features of colitis with discrete shallow
ulcers throughout, particularly in the rectosigmoid and
descending colon (54a). Stool microscopy is shown in
54b.

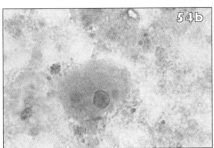

i. What is the diagnosis?
ii. Describe disease pathogenesis and
risk factors for this disorder.
iii. How may the diagnosis be
confirmed in suspected cases?
iv. Describe other gastrointestinal
manifestations of this disease.
v. Discuss treatment.

53 & 54: Answers

53 i. (e) Histamine may also bind to D-cells (on H3-receptors) to suppress somatostatin release. Acetylcholine is released from cholinergic nerves and binds to muscarinic receptors on the ECL cell to stimulate histamine release.
ii. (d) Gastrin release is responsible for up to 90% of the gastric phase of acid secretion.
iii. (b) A number of substances including prostaglandins, secretin, GIP (gastrin inhibitory peptide), peptide YY and somatostatin serve to inhibit parietal cell function and suppress acid secretion. Somatostatin is released by D-cells located in close histological association with G-cells and, thus, may act in a paracrine manner as a 'brake' on gastrin release.
iv. (a) The parietal cell is the primary functional unit responsible for gastric acid secretion. It contains multiple receptors on its basolateral membrane that are responsible for modulation of its function. Stimulatory receptors include those for gastrin (gastrin/CCK-B), histamine (H2), and acetylcholine (muscarinic/M3).
v. (c) The mucus neck cell secretes mucus and is the main source of bicarbonate secretion in the stomach.

54 i. Motile trophozoites in the stool with ingested red cells (**54b**) confirm invasive *Entamoeba histolytica* (amoebiasis).
ii. Ingestion of *E. histolytica* cysts, present in faecally contaminated material, initiates the infection. Excystation occurs in the bowel, and trophozoites are formed as a result of division of the cysts' nuclei. Trophozoites colonize the colon and produce cysts. In a minority of cases, *E. histolytica* adheres to the colon wall, induces an inflammatory reaction and becomes invasive. Amoebiasis is more common in developing countries, due to poor sanitation and overcrowding, and in the immunocompromised and institutionalized. It may be sexually transmitted.
iii. By finding motile trophozoites with ingested red cells in a fresh stool or on histology (**54c**).
iv. Manifestations of infection include asymptomatic non-invasive colonization (asymptomatic cyst passers); invasive colitis as demonstrated in this case; and chronic non-dysenteric intestinal amoebiasis which may mimic ulcerative colitis. Toxic

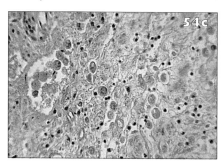

megacolon and perforation may occur, and a localized granulation response, producing a mass (amoeboma), may mimic a neoplasm. Stricturing may also occur. Approximately 10% of patients who have invasive amoebiasis develop an amoebic liver abscess.
v. Metronidazole is the therapy of choice; few patients require surgery for perforation or medical unresponsiveness.

55 A 72-year-old man presents with jaundice and weight loss.
i. Describe the ERCP findings (55a).
ii. What procedure has been performed (55b)?
iii. What is the most likely diagnosis?
iv. How may this diagnosis be confirmed?
v. What are the therapeutic options?

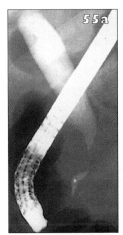 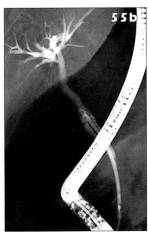

56 The chest radiograph (56a) was taken approximately 4 months before the CT scan (56b) in a patient who had originally presented with a hypochronic microcytic anaemia.
i. What does 56a demonstrate?
ii. What is the likely cause of the patient's anaemia?
iii. How may this condition be treated?
iv. What has happened in the 4-month gap between the two investigations?
v. What treatment may now be offered?

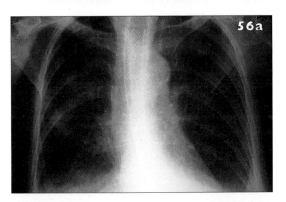

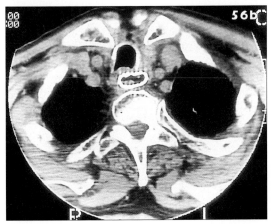

55 i. There is a stricture at the lower end of the common bile duct with dilatation of the common bile duct (**55a**).
ii. Endoscopic stent insertion into the common bile duct (**55b**).
iii. Carcinoma of the head of the pancreas.
iv. Abdominal ultrasound examination with ultrasound-guided needle biopsy of the pancreatic head. CT (± biopsy) of the pancreas may also be performed.
v. Surgery offers the only hope of cure, but fewer than 25% of tumours are potentially resectable, and only about 5% permit surgery with curative intent. In this case, a Whipple's type procedure is performed with resection of the tumour together with the distal stomach and duodenum. Pancreato-jejunostomy, choledochojejunostomy and gastrojejunostomy are required. The operative mortality is high, and careful preoperative staging is essential to minimize the number of inappropriate procedures. Endoscopic ultrasound is showing promise as a supplement to the information available from CT and MRI scanning. Radiotherapy has little role, but advances in chemotherapy suggest that useful palliation may be achieved. The most effective method of relieving obstructive jaundice in the incurable patient has been carefully investigated. The least invasive technique is the insertion of a biliary stent at ERCP, but there is a higher frequency of repeat procedures for stent blockage and duodenal obstruction than in patients receiving initial surgical bypass, who have a higher operative morbidity and mortality.

56 i. An oesophageal metal stent is present on the chest radiograph (**56a**).
ii. The placement of metal stents must be considered as permanent so their use is restricted to palliation of malignant tumours, bleeding from which is the cause of this patient's iron-deficient anaemia. Neither radiotherapy nor chemotherapy have an established role in the management of upper gastrointestinal adenocarcinomas. Surgery is best limited to tumours without mediastinal spread, as assessed by endoscopic ultrasonography. However, even in the absence of spread, 5-year survival is only 25% following surgery (<10% for unselected cases).
iii. Metal stents are placed endoscopically under fluoroscopic screening. The metal itself is protected by a gel and outer sheath that is withdrawn once positioned correctly to expose the gel to oesophageal secretions. The gel then dissolves allowing the stent to expand into position. Subsequent dilatation by balloon may help to ensure adequate luminal patency.
iv. The CT scan (**56b**) demonstrates the stent *in situ* but with evidence of tumour ingrowth, narrowing its lumen, a common occurrence with open mesh stents. Newer coated stents have reduced the incidence of complications.
v. As stents are narrowed by tumour growth or become invaded further balloon dilatation may help. Alternatively, ethanol may be injected to cause tumour necrosis. Laser may also reduce tumour bulk. Should these modalities fail, a second metal stent may be placed inside the first.

57 A 27-year-old man presented with a history of fresh haematemesis, having been out drinking with friends the night before. On admission he was not shocked and his haemoglobin was normal. Endoscopy was carried out 4 hours following admission (57).
i. What was the cause of the haematemesis?
ii. What is the pathophysiology of this condition?
iii. What is the prognosis?
iv. How would you treat this condition?

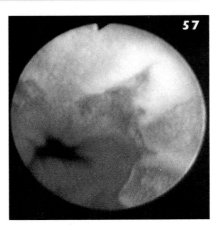

58 A 69-year-old man is brought to the emergency room with a history of vomiting copious amounts of blood that day. He is found to be cold and clammy with a pulse of 122/min and a systolic blood pressure of 84 mmHg. There is minimal epigastric tenderness. The rectal vault contains melanotic stool. The examination is otherwise unremarkable. He takes a 'baby' aspirin daily for ischaemic heart disease and a transient cerebral ischaemic episode that occurred 3 years previously. He uses an occasional over-the-counter H2-receptor antagonist for indigestion. He has mild glucose intolerance controlled by dietary measures. He smokes five cigarettes daily, but there is no history of alcoholism or liver disease. There is a strong family history of peptic ulcer disease. The initial haemoglobin is 11.9 g/dl, and platelet count $202 \times 10^9/l$ (202 000/mm^3). The BUN is 39.8 mmol/l (56 mg/dl). A gastric lavage reveals fresh and altered blood that does not clear. An upper endoscopy demonstrates the abnormality shown in 58.
i. Describe the initial emergency room management.
ii. Discuss the setting in which further management is best achieved.
iii. What is the significance of the initial haematological and biochemical results?
iv. What are the likely causes of the bleed?
v. Describe the endoscopic abnormality and its treatment.
vi. Discuss additional treatment issues.

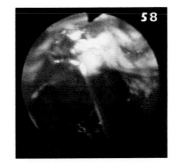

57 & 58: Answers

57 i. A Mallory–Weiss tear at the gastro-oesophageal junction.
ii. The cause is a longitudinal tearing of the cardiac mucosa, which is forced through the diaphragmatic hiatus during retching. A closed pylorus and retrograde propulsion of gastric contents in association with an increase in abdominal pressure generates high pressures in the proximal stomach which is then pushed through the diaphragmatic hiatus. There is usually a history of vomiting, retching, coughing or recent binge drinking.
iii. The condition originally described was thought rare but usually fatal. Endoscopy has, however, shown mucosal tears to be common, and over 90% of episodes resolve spontaneously.
iv. Resuscitation with appropriate replacement of blood and fluid loss are necessary. Endoscopy establishes the diagnosis. In a few cases, endoscopic haemostasis is necessary. Where this fails, balloon tamponade has been tried. Alternatives include angiographic embolization or vasopressin infusion. Rarely is surgery necessary.

58 i. Supporting the circulation must be given high priority in patients with severe GI haemorrhage. Venous access must be obtained and saline, volume expanders or blood transfused. Acid suppression is modestly beneficial. Establishing baseline renal, electrolyte, haematological and coagulation profiles facilitates later management decisions. Insertion of a nasogastric tube to evaluate on-going bleeding may assist in determining intervention, but is controversial. Lavage with iced saline is of no value and may be detrimental.
ii. Patients with on-going bleeding, who present or remain shocked, or who are at increased risk for an adverse outcome due to age or co-morbidity, are best managed in an intensive care unit.
iii. A normal or near-normal haemoglobin early after a bleed may lead to a false sense of security as haemodilution may take a few hours to occur. The elevated BUN suggests hypovolaemia or the intestinal absorption of blood.
iv. Over half of all cases of acute upper GI bleeding are caused by peptic ulceration or erosive disease. Aspirin and non-steroidal anti-inflammatory consumption is seen in 60% of patients admitted. Oesophageal varices are responsible for approximately 10% of cases. Mallory–Weiss tears, oesophagitis and vascular lesions account for the majority of the remainder. Tumours are rarely responsible.
v. Patients who present with shock, remain unstable despite resuscitation, continue to bleed, or who are at risk for varices, should be urgently investigated. This patient (58) demonstrates an actively bleeding (gastric) ulcer.
vi. Surgery would be necessary if endoscopic therapy fails to stop the bleeding, or if bleeding recurs. *Helicobacter pylori* status should be determined in patients with peptic ulceration. The ulcer should be treated medically for at least 6–8 weeks, and its benign nature and healing confirmed.

59 A 64-year-old man presents with a 2-month history of diarrhoea, haematochezia, and left lower quadrant abdominal pain. His haemoglobin is 11.0 g/dl. He denied any recent travel, antibiotic use, or contacts with persons with similar symptoms. His past medical history is unremarkable. Colonoscopy demonstrated inflammation of the rectum which extended to the mid-sigmoid colon where the erythema ended abruptly (59). The mucosa upstream of this was completely normal.

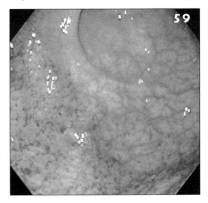

i. What is the probable diagnosis?
ii. Discuss the differential diagnosis.
iii. What tests are ordered for the evaluation?
iv. Comment on the pathological features of the most likely diagnosis.
v. Discuss possible therapy.

60 A 60-year-old woman complains of central abdominal pain, abdominal bloating, and vomiting food and bile, occurring 10–20 minutes after meals. Also in association with meals, she reports diarrhoea and occasional dizziness. She has become afraid to eat and has lost 9 kg (20 lb) since her symptoms began. The abdomen is soft and not distended. There is non-specific epigastric tenderness without any mass being palpated. She relates these symptoms to gastric surgery she underwent for an ulcer 5 years previously. The haemoglobin is 10.8 g/dl. An upper endoscopy demonstrates a solid ball of semi-digested 'food' and vegetable matter in a 10 cm gastric remnant (60). A widely patent anastomosis leading into two separate loops is seen. No ulceration is visualized.

i. Which surgical procedure was performed?
ii. What are the causes of pain and vomiting following this procedure?
iii. Comment on the diarrhoea and dizziness.
iv. What is the 'mass' visualized? Discuss the circumstances predisposing to its formation.
v. Discuss the causes of anaemia following gastric surgery.
vi. How would you manage this patient?

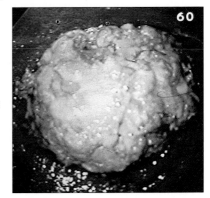

59 i. Ulcerative colitis.

ii. Inflammatory bowel disease in older persons is commonly mistaken for infectious colitis, ischaemic colitis and diverticulitis. While there is a bimodal incidence of inflammatory bowel disease (15–25 years and 55–65 years), the second peak is much smaller.

iii. Stool cultures, including testing for *Clostridium difficile*, and histology of colonic biopsies.

iv. In ulcerative colitis, colonic biopsies typically reveal crypt abscesses and a dense inflammatory infiltrate of the lamina propria, with goblet cell depletion and architectural distortion. Inflammation includes the rectum and extends proximally without skip lesions.

v. Most patients respond to oral or topical 5-aminosalicylic acid preparations. Steroid enemas may be utilized if the response is suboptimal. Oral corticosteroids are seldom required.

60 i. A Billroth II gastrectomy: distal gastric resection leading into an afferent (blind) loop into which pancreatic and biliary secretions drain, and into an efferent limb in continuity with the jejunum.

ii. Recurrent or anastomotic ulceration, luminal stenosis, bile gastritis, afferent and efferent loop syndromes, adhesions, and the dumping syndromes.

iii. There may be postvagotomy diarrhoea. The disconnection of pancreatic secretions and bile from the intestinal 'mainstream' may result in failure of nutrient–digestive enzyme mixing temporally – precipitating a malabsorption problem. In the early dumping syndrome, rapid emptying of hyperosmolar chyme into the small bowel occurs. The circulating blood volume is reduced due to secretion of fluid into the proximal intestine. Diarrhoea and some vasomotor symptoms may therefore occur 10–30 minutes following a meal. Late dumping symptoms arise from rapid glucose absorption, inappropriate insulin release, and late hypoglycaemia. Other mechanisms for diarrhoea include bacterial overgrowth in the afferent limb, and the unmasking of a latent gluten enteropathy.

iv. A bezoar – a mass of food or foreign material that has failed to clear the stomach because of altered gastric anatomy and motility.

v. Iron-deficiency anaemia is common following gastric resection. Gastric acid is important in the absorption of inorganic ferric iron. Maldigestion, reduced dietary intake and losses from bile gastritis aggravate the deficiency. Vitamin B_{12} levels may fall as a result of the loss of intrinsic factor and the absence of acid facilitation of digestion of food-bound vitamin B_{12}.

vi. Endoscopy to rule out a mechanical problem in the upper gastrointestinal tract is performed. If normal, a barium study is considered to examine the anatomical relationships and function of the loops and distal small bowel. Pancreatitis and biliary disease are excluded. Patients with dumping require a trial of dietary manipulation and efforts to delay gastric emptying. Octreotide may be useful if dietary measures fail. Remedial surgery is considered for those with debilitating symptoms unresponsive to the above.

61 A 60-year-old woman presented as an emergency with a haematemesis. She was shocked. Following initial assessment and resuscitation therapeutic endoscopic was performed. The patient's condition did not improve despite an apparently successful procedure and resuscitation measures. Urgent laparotomy was arranged (61).
i. What were the operative findings?
ii. What was the likely cause?
iii. How can the risk of this be minimized?

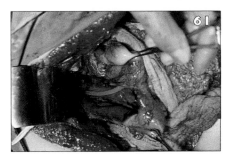

62 A 10-year-old girl presents with an 8-month history of crampy abdominal pain, weight loss and intermittent diarrhoea. Over the previous 6 weeks the pain has been more severe and constant, keeping her awake at night. The diarrhoea has increased in frequency and volume, and she has noticed small amounts of blood in the toilet water. She has had a reduced appetite, intermittent low-grade fevers and a documented lack of weight gain since she last visited the doctor 18 months previously. She also complains of arthralgias and a persistent mouth sore. On physical examination she is a thin girl with pale conjunctivae. Her gingival mucosa reveals lesions (62a). Her abdomen is soft with mild diffuse tenderness, especially over the right lower quadrant where there is a questionable fullness or mass. Rectal examination is normal but stool is positive for occult blood. Laboratory findings include a haemoglobin of 7.1 mg/dl, ESR of 45 mm/h and albumin of 22 g/l. Stool culture, ova and parasite examination and *Clostridium difficile* toxin assay are all negative.
i. What diagnosis is most likely?
ii. How would you proceed with the evaluation?
iii. What may the abdominal mass indicate, and how may this be confirmed?
iv. Describe how this entity affects children differently from adults.
v. Discuss treatment of this entity in children.

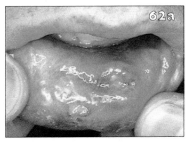

61 & 62: Answers

61 i. Full-thickness necrosis and perforation of the stomach wall.
ii. A complication of injection of sclerosant, possibly compounded by relative hypotension and hypoxia.
iii. It is essential to use the lowest feasible volume of a dilute and well-placed sclerosant. Successful haemostasis also is reported with epinephrine (adrenaline) alone diluted to 1 in 100 000. The patient should be well resuscitated before the procedure, and oxygen given to reduce the magnitude of hypoxia.

62 i. Crohn's disease.
ii. Biopsy of the gingival lesion may reveal typical non-caseating granulomatous changes. Radiographic contrast studies may demonstrate characteristic areas of narrowed or inflamed and ulcerated bowel – which may be viewed directly endoscopically at colonoscopy with ileoscopy (**62b**). Definitive diagnosis requires the presence of granulomas on biopsy (**62c**).

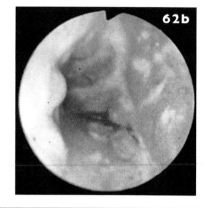

iii. Thickened and inflamed bowel wall and mesentery in the region of the terminal ileum. However, an abscess due to fistulization or perforation is also possible. Abdominal CT with contrast is often useful (**62d**).
iv. Disease limited to the colon is less common. Growth retardation may precede clinical symptoms by years with impaired linear growth being present in approximately half of children at the time of diagnosis, which tends to be more delayed than in adults.

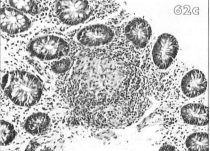

v. Therapy is similar to that for adult Crohn's disease except that to maintain adequate growth and nutrition is a more major focus of treatment. Permanent short stature affects up to 25% of patients who have the disease before puberty.

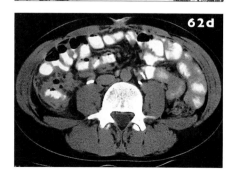

63 A 65-year-old man was found to be anaemic during work-up for a routine cataract operation. Apart from deteriorating vision he was asymptomatic. Faecal occult bloods were consistently positive and an upper GI endoscopy was normal. Colonoscopy revealed multiple lesions (63).
i. What is the diagnosis?
ii. What other investigation may be useful in diagnosing this condition?
iii. What treatment is available?

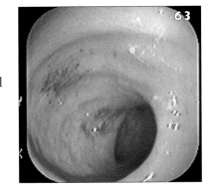

64 A 25-year-old man carries the diagnosis of irritable bowel syndrome because of several months of complaints of loose voluminous stool and colicky abdominal pain. The abdominal pain has recently increased in intensity. Other complaints include diffuse mild joint stiffness and pain, especially of the knees and lower back. Physical examination reveals moderate tenderness and a sense of fullness in the right lower quadrant. Flexible sigmoidoscopy is normal. The ESR rate is 82 mm/h. The patient undergoes a small-bowel follow-through radiography (64a and 64b).
i. What is the diagnosis?
ii. Describe the radiological abnormalities.
iii. What further testing may be necessary?
iv. Is a surgical approach for this finding warranted?
v. What other diseases produce stricturing of the terminal ileum?

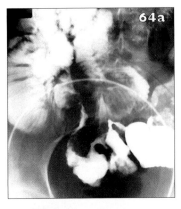

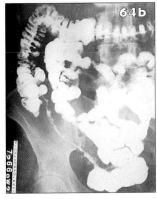

63 & 64: Answers

63 i. The diagnosis is angiodysplasia. These cherry-red, fern-like vascular malformations are often multiple, and are found most frequently in the right colon of patients aged over 60 years. There is an association with chronic renal failure and also with aortic stenosis. The lesions consist of dilated, tortuous, submucosal vessels and in severe cases the mucosa may be replaced by a mass of dilated, deformed vessels.
ii. The two investigations useful in the diagnosis of this condition are colonoscopy and angiography. Selective angiography of the mesenteric arteries using subtraction techniques may show densely opacified, dilated, tortuous, slow-emptying intramural veins and associated clusters of slow-emptying vessels seen during the arterial phase. Early filling of veins, visualized within 6–8 s, is very suggestive of angiodysplasia and probably arises from the development of arteriovenous communications.
iii. Indications for treatment in angiodysplasia are bleeding requiring blood transfusion, or persistent anaemia despite iron-replacement therapy. Isolated lesions can be ablated with endoscopic thermal or laser therapy. If this cannot be performed, or fails, surgical resection is appropriate, providing that there is confidence in the site of bleeding. If neither are effective, oestrogen–progesterone therapy can be tried – some success has been reported therewith.

64 i. Crohn's disease involving the terminal ileum.
ii. The mucosal pattern of the terminal ileum is irregular and ulcerated. There is asymmetric dilatation of a segment upstream of a narrowed area. A long stricture is present in the distal ileum, the so-called string sign. Although the radiological abnormalities may be marked, correlation with symptoms is highly variable.
iii. The diagnosis may be confirmed by colonoscopy and intubation of the ileocaecal valve with biopsy of obvious abnormalities. The caecum is abnormal in more than half of subjects with Crohn's disease of the terminal ileum. Vitamin B_{12} levels may be low in patients with extensive ileal disease.
iv. Therapy is individualized. Approximately one-third of patients with Crohn's disease undergo surgery at some stage. More than one-half of these individuals require repeat surgical intervention, often to deal with recurrent disease, fistulae or strictures that frequently complicate the initial procedure. The majority of patients with symptomatic terminal ileal disease, however, respond to medical therapy consisting of either or a combination of a 5-aminosalicylic acid preparation [sulfapyridine or mesalamine (mesalazine)], antimicrobials or oral corticosteroids. Occasionally, an immunosuppressive agent may be necessary. Hospitalization and resection are required for patients who do not respond to medical therapy or who develop intestinal obstruction. Short strictures situated in the terminal ileum may be amenable to endoscopic dilation.
v. Other diseases that may cause a similar radiological appearance include lymphoma, tuberculosis, carcinoid, radiation, NSAID-related enteritis and adenocarcinoma.

65 A 25-year-old man is admitted to the emergency room with a gunshot wound in the abdomen. It is unclear as to when precisely the incident occurred. At laparotomy, the bullet is found to have transected the superior mesenteric artery, which cannot be repaired. The greater part of the small intestine is already necrotic. A massive small-intestinal resection is performed. The duodenum is anastomosed to the right colon.
i. What are the most common conditions that necessitate the resection of massive sections of the small intestine?
ii. Comment on the expected postoperative symptoms that these patients may experience.
iii. Which nutritional deficiencies may be anticipated?
iv. Comment on the potential risk of renal calculi.
v. Comment on the potential risk of gallstones.

66 A 58-year-old man with lifelong constipation and several years' abdominal pain was further investigated. On five occasions in the preceding 3 years he had been admitted to another hospital with apparent intestinal obstruction. On one of these admissions an exploratory laparotomy had been performed with no abnormality found. Repeated barium studies and endoscopies of the upper and lower bowel had failed to provide an explanation. There was an additional past history of recurrent urinary tract infections. Investigation of these had revealed an enlarged atonic bladder with unilateral megaureter and hydronephrosis. Shown are the barium follow-through (66a) and barium meal (66b).

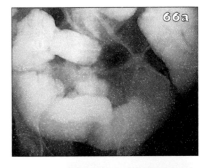

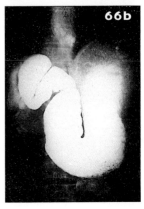

i. What are the key abnormalities in the two films?
ii. What is the likely diagnosis?
iii. What other medical conditions are considered in a patient such as this?
iv. In the absence of an underlying systemic condition, what is expected histologically?
v. This man occasionally had problematic diarrhoea and flatulence. Why might this be and what can be done about it?

65 i. The most common causes of major small-intestinal loss include acute mesenteric artery ischaemia, thrombosis of the superior mesenteric vein, and vascular compromise due to small intestinal volvulus and strangulated internal or external hernias. Multiple intestinal resections in the setting of Crohn's and radiation bowel disease may also lead to a short-bowel syndrome. Neonates with necrotizing enterocolitis may need massive resection.

ii. Resection of the small intestine reduces the surface area available for absorption of ingested nutrients and physiological secretions. Disabling, life-threatening diarrhoea resulting in dehydration and electrolyte disturbances is common. Malabsorption may be severe. Bacterial overgrowth frequently occurs. Acid peptic disease may develop secondary to hypergastrinaemia.

iii. Major resections of the small intestine place increases the risk for dehydration, calorie and nutrient malabsorption and losses. Loss of the terminal ileum depletes the bile salt pool, resulting in malabsorption of fat and fat-soluble vitamins A, D, E and K. Also, ileal resection impairs absorption of vitamin B_{12}. Calcium deficiency may occur secondary to vitamin D deficiency. Zinc and magnesium deficiencies are often seen.

iv. Dietary oxalate binds to calcium in the intestinal lumen. Calcium complexed with unabsorbed fatty acids increases the opportunity for oxalate to be absorbed by both the small and large intestines. Absorbed oxalate may complex with calcium and predispose to renal stones. Stones are also more likely by continual dehydration.

v. Diminution of the bile salt pool results in a relative increase in the biliary cholesterol concentration, facilitating the formation of a supersaturated bile, setting the stage for gallstone formation.

66 i. Small-bowel follow-through (**66a**) demonstrates a grossly dilated small bowel with loss of characteristic valvulae coniventes. Barium meal (**66b**) shows gastric stasis and megaduodenum.

ii. Chronic idiopathic intestinal pseudo-obstruction (CIIP).

iii. Visceral myopathies; amyloidosis; connective tissue diseases (dermatomyositis, polymyositis, systemic sclerosis, SLE); muscular dystrophies; diabetes mellitus; hypothyroidism; acute intermittent porphyria; phaeochromocytoma; brainstem strokes; Parkinson's disease; spinal cord injury; Chagas' disease; vinca alkaloids; tricyclic antidepressants; phenothiazines; opiates; visceral neuropathies (sporadic/familial developmental abnormalities).

iv. Idiopathic causes of chronic intestinal pseudo-obstruction include the visceral myopathies and neuropathies. All the former are characterized by fibrosis, muscle atrophy and vacuolation with degeneration of the muscularis propria. In contrast, the changes of systemic sclerosis do not typically cause vacuolar degeneration but are characterized by progressive fibrosis.

Sporadic visceral myopathies include degenerative disorders of the submucosal and myenteric plexi; degeneration may be seen in axons, dendrites and neurones and may be associated with inflammatory changes.

v. Bacterial overgrowth; treatment with antibiotics may help alleviate some symptoms such as diarrhoea, abdominal pain and bloating. Many patients need rotating courses of antibiotics for 1 week each month to keep symptoms at bay.

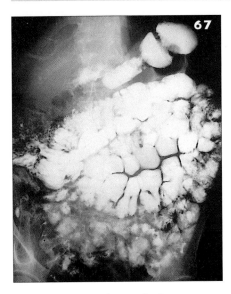

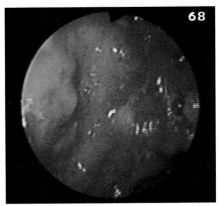

68 Shown (68) is the terminal ileum seen at colonoscopy in a patient with diarrhoea and weight loss.
i. Describe the appearances in 68.
ii. What are the differential diagnoses?
iii. What other investigations may be indicated?
iv. How should this patient be treated?
v. What is the prognosis?

67 A patient with Marfan's syndrome presented with diarrhoea and weight loss (67).
i. What is the radiological diagnosis?
ii. What is the most likely cause of his symptoms?

69 A 5-year-old girl has been noted to have had fresh rectal bleeding for 3 months. Stools are soft but formed. Occasional crampy abdominal pain has occurred. She is growing normally and has an excellent appetite. There is no family history of gastrointestinal disease. Examination is normal with no abnormalities of the skin or anal fissure. Sigmoidoscopy demonstrated the lesion seen in 69a.
i. What is the probable diagnosis?
ii. Describe its frequency and usual presentation.
iii. Describe the pathological features usually present.
iv. Discuss alternative diagnoses possible for the presentation described.
v. How should you proceed with diagnosis and therapy?

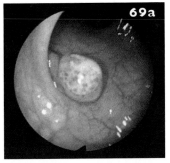

67 i. Jejunal diverticulosis.
ii. Secondary bacterial overgrowth.

68 i. The terminal ileum is markedly nodular, but there is no ulceration and the mucosal surface is essentially normal.
ii. Immune deficiency states that result in small intestinal nodular lymphoid hyperplasia:
- Selective IgA deficiency, in which increased mucosal IgM production compensates for IgA lack, and the expanded population of IgM-secreting B-cells appears as submucous nodularity. Such individuals are usually asymptomatic.
- Variable acquired immunoglobulin deficiency, a heterogeneous syndrome of B-cell maturation defects. There are decreased numbers of plasma cells in the lamina propria, and large lymphoid follicles throughout the small intestine, often with villous stunting or total villous atrophy. The symptomatology makes this deficiency more likely.
- Nodular lymphoid hyperplasia – this has also been described in apparently normal individuals.

iii. Measurement of serum immunoglobulins, barium follow-through and jejunal biopsies. Bacterial overgrowth may also be demonstrable with vitamin B_{12} malabsorption.
iv. Normal human immunoglobulin is given intravenously every 4 weeks. The dose is adjusted until the patient remains free from infection.
v. The prognosis is good, and long-term survival is expected.

69 i. Juvenile polyp.
ii. Juvenile polyp is the most common type of intestinal tumour in childhood occurring in up to 1% of pre-school children. Juvenile polyps account for 90% of colorectal polyps in children and are usually diagnosed between 2 and 10 years of age. Children with juvenile polyps usually present with painless, mild haematochezia. Occasionally, bleeding may be profuse. Other symptoms include intermittent crampy abdominal pain, anaemia, rectal prolapse or intussusception. Over 25% of children with one polyp have a second polyp elsewhere in the colon. If a child has more than five polyps, a polyposis syndrome is likely.
iii. Juvenile polyps are hamartomas and consist of a cluster of mucoid lakes

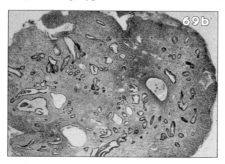

surrounded by mucus-secreting glandular cells (**69b**). They are usually large (0.5–3 cm) and pedunculated.
iv. Other diagnoses include solitary rectal ulcer or haemangioma. Anal fissure is usually painful.
v. Diagnosis is best accomplished by endoscopic examination with polypectomy. Unless an individual has a polyposis syndrome, the risk of carcinoma is remote.

70 A 71-year-old man seeks evaluation of bright red rectal bleeding and anaemia. Two years previously he received a curative course of radiotherapy for prostate cancer. His stools are loose and he has daily rectal pain. He has received six units of packed red cells over the past 3 months. Laboratory tests include haemoglobin 9.8 g/dl; MCV 71 fl; and negative stool culture. Flexible sigmoidoscopy reveals poorly compliant, pale rectal mucosa with telangiectasia (70).

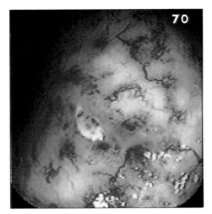

i. What is the diagnosis?
ii. Comment on the pathophysiology of this disorder.
iii. Which complications may occur?
iv. Comment on therapeutic options.
v. What is the role of surgery in this disorder?

71 A 69-year-old man with a history of depression develops abdominal distension 2 days following a coronary artery bypass grafting procedure. The operation was not complicated by undue hypotension or arrhythmias. He complains of mild abdominal discomfort and dyspnoea. He has not passed stool or flatus since the surgery. He is afebrile and haemodynamically stable. The abdomen is distended and tympanic with high-pitched bowel sounds. There is no peritonism. The rectal vault is empty. There are no abdominal scars and the hernial sites are intact. He has a WBC count of 12×10^9/l (12 000/mm^3) and haemoglobin of 14.3 g/dl. Radiology demonstrates bilateral basal atelectasis (mild), and massive dilatation of the colon (71a). There is air in the rectum but the caecum is 15 cm in diameter and there is a lack of haustration in the right colon. The small bowel is slightly dilated.

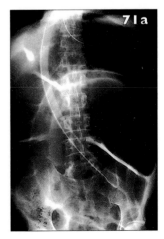

i. What is the likely diagnosis?
ii. Discuss other diagnostic possibilities.
iii. What additional investigations may be helpful?
iv. Comment on the potential complications that may occur.
v. Describe treatment of this disorder.

70 i. Radiation proctitis.

ii. Injury is most common following radiotherapy to the prostate, cervix, uterus and bladder, and most commonly affects organs that are generally immobile due to intrinsic fixation or adhesions immobilizing loops of ileum in the radiation beam. Acute radiation injury is immediate and results in transient diarrhoea and urgency, while the chronic form of injury is delayed months to years and results in diarrhoea, rectal bleeding and rectal pain due to a radiation-induced obliterative arteritis.

iii. Proctosigmoiditis with recurrent bleeding, ulceration, fistulization (mainly rectovesical, rectovaginal) and stricturing may occur.

iv. Although mild cases may spontaneously remit, most do not, and conventional therapy is ineffective. Laser photocoagulation, however, is promising and surgery is rarely appropriate.

v. There is a high complication rate due to the relative hypovascularity of the tissues involved. Wound dehiscence and infections are common. A diverting colostomy is sometimes required.

71 i. Acute, colonic pseudo-obstruction (Ogilvie's syndrome).

ii. Other potential causes include ischaemic colitis, toxic megacolon in association with inflammatory bowel disease, retroperitoneal haemorrhage, uraemia, metabolic abnormalities (e.g. hypothyroidism) and drugs (e.g. antidepressants). A primary form occurs as part of a visceral neuropathy or myopathy.

iii. Radiography of the abdomen is performed to exclude perforation. A water-soluble contrast examination excludes any stenotic lesions of the colon. A blood count, serum potassium, magnesium, calcium, renal profile and TSH are requested.

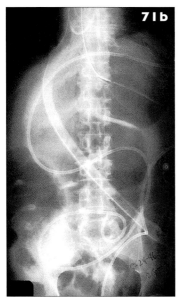

71b

iv. Colonic perforation is the most feared complication, occurring in 15% of cases with a mortality rate of over 40%. Patients are also at risk for vomiting and pulmonary aspiration.

v. Electrolyte and fluid disturbances must be corrected. Nasogastric and rectal tube placement may be useful. Up to 30% of patients improve with conservative measures. Rolling the patient and prokinetic agents may be effective. Colonoscopy permits air removal by suctioning during the withdrawal phase. To avoid recurrence, a colon decompression tube may be inserted (71b). Surgery is reserved for failure of colonoscopic decompression, or for perforation.

72 A middle-aged man presents with motor neurone disease.
i What has happened?
ii. For which other patient groups might such a procedure be appropriate? What contraindications apply?
iii. What are the main complications?

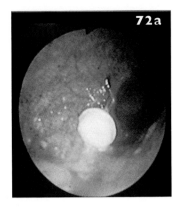

73 A 61-year-old carpenter presents with persistent upper abdominal pain, aggravated by food, and early satiety. He has vomited intermittently and has noticed blood in the vomitus on at least one occasion. He has lost approximately 9 kg (20 lb) in weight over a 3-month period. On physical examination a firm mass is palpable in the epigastrium. Firm lymph nodes are present in both supraclavicular fossae. A complete blood count reveals a haemoglobin of 9.8 g/dl; MCV 72 fl; platelets 97×10^9/l (97 000/mm³); albumin 36 g/l; and ALP 284 u/l (normal <110 u/l). A barium meal demonstrates an antral abnormality (73a) and at endoscopy a friable, ulcerated mass lesion involving the gastric antrum is seen (73b).

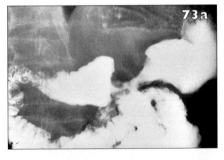

i. What is the likely diagnosis?
ii. Explain the abnormal haematological and biochemical results.
iii. What additional investigations may be necessary?
iv. Describe precursor conditions for this disease.
v. Discuss treatment modalities.

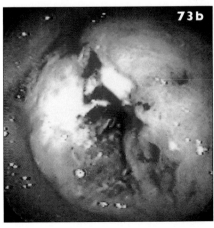

72 & 73: Answers

72 i. He has had a PEG tube inserted; it is secured with a buffer retaining it on the intraluminal side (72b).
ii. PEG tube insertion provides a convenient and reliable means of enteral feeding and is the preferred method for those whose need for nutritional support is likely to persist for 30 days or more and in whom the enteral route is usable, including those with neurological impairment or inability to swallow, following stroke, multiple sclerosis, obstructing lesions in the oropharynx, or major facial burns.

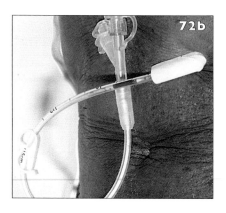

Relative contraindications include: ascites; portal hypertension; coagulopathy; gastric outflow obstruction; active gastric ulceration; abdominal wall infection; peritoneal dialysis; and those in whom endoscopy is not possible (when a radiologically guided percutaneous method may be considered).
iii. Complications are those of endoscopy, i.e. visceral perforation and procedure-related sepsis, and those related to intragastric feeding, such as aspiration and tube blockage; altered body image may also cause morbidity.

73 i. Adenocarcinoma of the gastric antrum.
ii. The anaemia is the result of blood loss, chronic disease and poor nutrition. A tumour-related microangiopathic haemolytic anaemia may also occur. The thrombocytopenia may be due to this or to marantic endocarditis, which can be a terminal event in disseminated mucinous adenocarcinomatosis. The elevated alkaline phosphatase suggests liver metastases.
iii. Gastric histology and endoscopic ultrasonography, which is more sensitive than CT scanning. The latter plays a vital role in the evaluation of the probable distant spread.
iv. Chronic atrophic gastritis and intestinal metaplasia are most closely linked to an increased risk of gastric cancer. H. pylori is strongly implicated. Meta-analyses suggest that partial gastrectomy is associated with a 1.5- to three-fold risk beginning 15–20 years after resection. Pernicious anaemia is associated with an up to three-fold excess risk of stomach cancer. Other precursor lesions include Ménétrier's disease and gastric adenomatous polyps. The rise in the incidence of proximal carcinoma may be related to an increasing incidence of Barrett's oesophagus. Familial syndromes have been described.
v. Surgery offers the only chance of cure. Bypass of obstructing lesions provides symptomatic, but transient relief. Endoscopic laser therapy and stenting are useful in specific circumstances. The value of radiotherapy remains uncertain. Chemotherapy produces reasonable palliation, but median survival ranges from 6 to 10 months.

74 An obese 38-year-old woman presented with intolerable epigastric and retrosternal chest pains. The pain was present constantly but exacerbated by bending down and by swallowing hot or spicy food. An endoscopy was performed (74).
i. What is shown?
ii. Could the above findings be consistent with the symptoms?
iii. What treatment options are available?

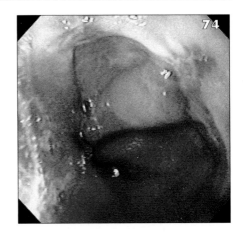

75 A 38-year-old businessman from Portugal had a 2-year history of the passage of 3–5 liquid stools per day, but no blood or mucus. He had lost 12 kg (26 lb) in the preceding 9 months. Initial benefit from loperamide was not maintained and he has urge faecal incontinence. He also describes tingling in the hands and feet which has become steadily more marked. He has had erectile impotence for 6 months. All his family live in Portugal. His younger brother required heart transplantation for cardiac failure in the previous year. His sister has been wheelchair-bound since the age of 33, his father died of heart failure at the age of 38 and two paternal uncles, also wheelchair-bound, have bowel and neurological complaints. The patient has two sons, aged 5 and 7, who are currently well. Routine haematological and biochemical tests are normal, but vitamin B_{12} level is low, and both CRP and ESR are about three times the upper limit of normal. 75 shows his barium follow-through. Upper GI endoscopy was macroscopically normal.

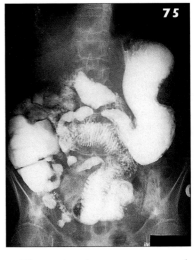

i. What is the likely diagnosis?
ii. What is the definitive investigation?

74 & 75: Answers

74 i. Shown in 74 is the oesophagogastric junction with a tongue of gastric mucosa extending caudally, consistent with mild oesophagitis.
ii. Yes. Symptoms of oesophagitis are extremely variable and do not correspond to the severity of the underlying inflammation. Often, the pain causes anorexia, weight loss and/or dysphagia. Swallowing difficulties may be caused by the pain or because of stricture formation. As oesophagitis is associated with reflux the presenting complaint may be of acid or food regurgitation.
iii. Simple lifestyle changes may ameliorate the symptoms. These include weight loss, stopping smoking, avoidance of acidic or spicy food, and reducing alcohol intake and caffeine-containing drinks. Sometimes, raising the head of the bed prevents acid reflux, as does avoiding eating just before bedtime.

Alginates are useful as they form a layer over the stomach contents, reducing reflux. This layer forms best in a non-acidic environment, rationalizing the combined use of alginates with acid suppressants.

Prokinetic agents increase the rate at which the stomach empties; cisapride increases the tone of the lower oesophageal sphincter.

Both H_2 receptor antagonists and proton pump inhibitors reduce, to various degrees, the amount of acid produced and remove the precipitant of reflux oesophagitis.

If medical therapy fails or the patient does not wish to take medicines for many years, surgery may be considered. The objective of all the various operations described is to increase the length of the abdominal oesophagus slightly and to improve the sphincteric action of the lower oesophagus. Sometimes, a diaphragmatic crural repair is done to prevent herniation of the stomach into the thoracic cavity. The most popular procedure is the Nissen fundoplication, now frequently carried out as a laparoscopic procedure.

75 i. He has familial amyloidosis with polyneuropathy. This is an autosomal dominant condition with variable penetrance. The diagnosis can be confirmed by demonstration of amyloid in any of the affected tissues (in this case on an endoscopically obtained distal duodenal biopsy). The changes on barium follow-through are not diagnostic. Screening by detection of abnormal variants of serum transthyretin is possible in asymptomatic relatives, but prenatal diagnosis is not yet possible.
ii. Autonomic neuropathy is common, as well as peripheral neuropathy, and this may contribute to the gastrointestinal features, as may secondary small-bowel bacterial overgrowth. Infiltration of the muscle of the anal sphincters and their denervation contribute to a high risk of faecal incontinence as the disease progresses.

There is no established therapy, but liver transplantation appears the most promising given that the disease probably results from hepatic production of an abnormal pre-albumin variant which has amyloidogenic properties. It is uncertain whether transplantation can reverse abnormalities that have already occurred. Without transplantation, death usually occurs from cardiac failure within 10 years of the first symptom.

76 An 8-year-old girl presented to the emergency department with a 36-hour history of vomiting. There was no bile in the vomitus, but there had been occasional streaks of fresh blood. The vomiting started in the early morning with no obvious precipitating factor. She reported having a headache and abdominal pain since the onset of the vomiting. There was no contact history with others with gastrointestinal symptoms. She had two similar episodes 6 weeks and 4 months previously for which admission and intravenous rehydration had been required. She was otherwise well with no relevant past history and she claimed to enjoy school, where her academic achievement was satisfactory. There was a family history only of irritable bowel syndrome. On examination, she was estimated to be 5–10% dehydrated, with mild epigastric tenderness. Initial investigation revealed a serum sodium level of 143 mmol/l and a bicarbonate level of 18 mmol/l, but was otherwise normal. During a further 3 days of vomiting intravenous rehydration was continued. She then appeared to make a complete recovery without specific therapy.
i. Name the most likely diagnosis.
ii. Name the principles of management to be applied.

77 Six months after being involved in a motor vehicle accident (he fell asleep at the wheel and ran into a tree), a 25-year-old man presents with a history of two attacks of acute pancreatitis, 1 month apart. He sustained light bruising to the chest and abdomen at the time of the accident, but radiographs were normal and he did not require hospitalization. He denies any alcoholism. Physical examination demonstrates tenderness to deep palpation in the left upper quadrant and epigastrium, but is otherwise unremarkable. He is haemodynamically stable with a normal blood count and liver enzymes. The serum amylase and lipase were both elevated during his previous episodes and are now near normal. Abdominal sonography of the upper abdomen is normal, but some air-filled bowel loops overlie the pancreas. A procedure is performed (77).

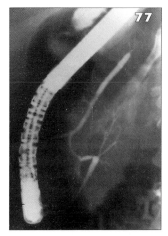

i. What does 77 show and what procedure is illustrated?
ii. What abnormality is demonstrated?
iii. What is the likely cause of this finding ?
iv. What is the preferred management?
v. What additional radiological investigation is appropriate?

76 & 77: Answers

76 i. Although a posterior fossa tumour, peptic ulceration, intermittent intestinal obstruction from volvulus or malrotation, and metabolic conditions such as the urea cycle disorders, defects of organic acid handling, infective causes, intoxication such as in Munchausen-by-proxy, and Addison's disease, should be considered, the most likely diagnosis is cyclical vomiting syndrome (CVS). Though a little more common than most of the above, CVS unfortunately remains a diagnosis of exclusion. It is therefore necessary to exclude infection, intracranial lesions, metabolic pathology, and structural abnormalities of the upper gastrointestinal tract. CVS is not well understood. Affected patients usually feel well between episodes and have no prodrome. Vomiting often lasts for several days and then stops spontaneously or with antiemetic therapy. Intervals between episodes vary from a few weeks to over a year, but CVS is benign and often resolves with increasing age.
ii. Management is supportive with fluids and antiemetics given as necessary. Early use of ondansetron may be particularly helpful.

77 i. Pancreatogram by the injection of contrast retrogradely up the pancreatic duct via the papilla of Vater. The procedure is endoscopic retrograde cholangiopancreatography (ERCP) (77). The lower part of the endoscope is also seen.
ii. Abrupt and premature termination of the pancreatic duct in the mid-gland (body) region, presumably by a stricture. Secondary ducts of normal appearance are visualized in the head of the pancreas.
iii. This is the classic site of post-traumatic injury to the pancreatic duct associated with steering wheel injury; the force of the injury is transmitted through the gland, which lies across the spine. The duct is literally 'fractured', resulting in leakage of pancreatic fluid into the peritoneal cavity or communicating cystic cavity.
iv. When ductal injury is associated with recurrent pancreatitis or fistula formation, surgical resection of the affected part of the pancreas is almost always required. Occasionally it may be possible to place a stent (prosthesis) endoscopically over the leak to bridge the gap across the severed duct, which may promote healing and restitution of normal pancreatic flow. This is best performed very early but is not always feasible, even in the most skillful of hands. Pancreatic duct strictures may also be amenable to endoscopic-assisted dilatation. Long-term follow-up results of these procedures remain anecdotal.
v. An abdominal CT scan should be performed to look for additional pancreatic pathology, including pseudocyst formation.

78 A 60-year-old male presented with retrosternal discomfort. His family doctor requested this barium meal (78).
i. What is the diagnosis?
ii. What are the major complications?
iii. What is Borchardt's triad?
iv. What treatment is indicated?

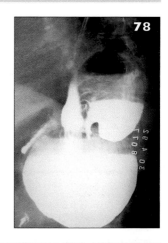

79 A 46-year-old woman presents with a 5-month history of dysphagia for solids and liquids, regurgitation of partially undigested food, and intermittent cough. Previously, the patient had reported symptoms of heartburn and indigestion and was placed on omeprazole, 20 mg/day, with some improvement. The patient also reports a 7 kg (15 lb) weight loss over this period of time. She smokes 10 cigarettes a day. There is no history of foreign travel or Raynaud's phenomenon. On examination, the only notable feature was obesity. A chest radiograph (79a) and barium swallow (79b) are performed.

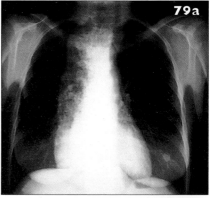

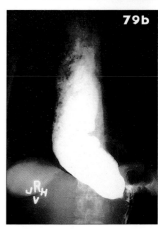

i. Which disorders does the history suggest?
ii. What investigations should be performed?
iii. Comment on the radiological features.
iv. What additional testing would be appropriate to confirm the diagnosis?
v. What is the pathogenesis of this problem?
vi. What are the therapeutic options for this problem?

71

78 & 79: Answers

78 i. This is a para-oesophageal or rolling hiatus hernia (**78**).
ii. It may be responsible for bleeding, gastric volvulus or strangulation.
iii. Borchardt's triad in gastric volvulus is that of severe epigastric pain, retching with an inability to vomit and difficulty in the passage of a nasogastric tube.
iv. Surgery is usually advised.

The para-oesophageal hernia is quite different from the much more common sliding hernia. It is usually seen late in life and often is associated with only vague symptoms until a major complication ensues. It is easier to diagnose radiologically than at endoscopy, and may be apparent at plain chest radiography where a gas bubble is seen adjacent to the oesophagus in the lower mediastinum. Owing to the severity of the potential complications and their relative frequency (akin to the risk of strangulation of a femoral hernia), surgery should be offered to all but the most frail.

79 i. (i) Benign oesophageal stricture secondary to reflux oesophagitis; (ii) carcinoma of the oesophagus; (iii) achalasia of the oesophagus; (iv) infectious oesophagitis; (v) scleroderma; (vi) extrinsic oesophageal compression.
ii. Barium oesophagogram with videofluoroscopic evaluation of swallowing for morphological and motor disorders. Endoscopy may help identify mucosal disease. Chest radiography or CT scan may be useful. Oesophageal manometry is indicated in some.
iii. The oesophagus is massively dilated and contains food debris. A smooth narrowing occurs at the level of the gastro-oesophageal junction, with retention of barium. The gastro-oesophageal junction appears intact without stricture or mass. This is achalasia.
iv. Oesophageal manometry may confirms achalasia (**79c**), demonstrating that lower oesophageal sphincter pressure is elevated and fails to relax completely with swallowing.

v. A loss of the inhibitory intrinsic nerves in the myenteric plexus results from depletion of nitric oxide synthase neurones in the myenteric plexus with preservation of cholinergic neurones.
vi. Nitrates or calcium channel blockers may provide transient relief but less than endoscopic balloon dilatation of the lower oesophageal sphincter. Laparoscopic surgical myotomy (Heller's myotomy) is an option. Botulinum toxin injection is also useful.

72

80 A 67-year-old woman presented with an acute episode of haematemesis.
She was shocked on admission (blood pressure 60/30 mmHg; pulse 110
beats/min) and had a haemoglobin of
8.4 g/dl. Endoscopy (80) was carried
out within 4 hours of admission.
There was fresh blood in the stomach
on endoscopy.
i. What is the vascular lesion shown
in 80?
ii. What other vascular lesions may
cause acute upper gastrointestinal
bleeding?
iii. How should this case be
managed?

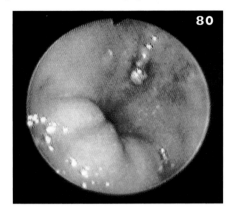

81 A 16-month-old infant presents to the paediatric surgeon with recurrent
rectal prolapse (81a), prior to which his developmental history was normal.
He was initially breast-fed and started on puréed, then solid, foods at expected
ages. He now has a voracious appetite, often eating 'man-sized' portions.
Despite the large food intake, weight, length and head circumference
monitoring demonstrate poor growth (81b). He has had large bowel
movements with soft stools, which are described as very foul smelling.
i. Describe the various forms of rectal prolapse.
ii. In which circumstances may prolapse occur?
iii. How is prolapse best treated?
iv. Which cause of growth disturbance is suggested by
the growth charts (81b)?
v. What additional diagnoses and tests should now be
considered?

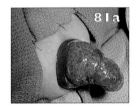

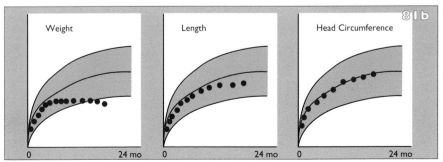

80 & 81: Answers

80 i. Dieulafoy's lesion (80), an ectatic submucosal artery which has eroded through the gastric mucosa and ruptured to cause bleeding.
ii. Other potential lesions include hereditary haemorrhagic telangiectasia, CRST syndrome, angiodysplasia, the water-melon stomach (gastric antral vascular ectasias), and arteriovenous malformations.
iii. Treatment may be possible endoscopically with injection sclerotherapy or bipolar coagulation, although surgery is often necessary.

81 i. Rectal prolapse implies protrusion of the rectum through the anus. Mucosal prolapse is most commonly found. Brief prolapse of a small amount of rectum is common with normal defaecation, but prolapse that includes the muscular and serosal layers (procidentia) is rare in childhood.
ii. It occurs most commonly in children aged under 2 years; the relatively flat infant sacrum and weak pelvic floor muscles probably are predisposing factors. Most cases occur in association with straining due to constipation, but also in cystic fibrosis or coeliac disease.
iii. Most reduce spontaneously. Occasionally, manual assistance is required. The prolapsed mucosa may bleed due to vascular congestion. Surgery may be required if the prolapse cannot be reduced, but treatment of underlying constipation or of an associated malabsorptive condition usually suffices.
iv. The growth charts shows that the rate of weight gain levelled off at 4–6 months. Linear growth decreased to a lesser degree and at an older age. Head growth remains normal. This is consistent with suboptimal caloric supply due to inadequate intake or malabsorption. A voracious appetite and foul-smelling stool suggests malabsorption.
v. Tests for malabsorptive disorders are obtained, beginning with a sweat test for cystic fibrosis. If inadequate sweat is obtained, DNA testing may confirm the diagnosis. Coeliac disease is also considered. In Western cultures, most infants consume gluten-containing cereals before 6 months of age, and symptoms of malabsorption typically ensue then. Screening antibody tests lack adequate sensitivity and specificity at this age. A small-bowel biopsy is therefore performed. In coeliac disease the biopsy reveals villous atrophy, crypt hyperplasia and an increased density of intraepithelial lymphocytes (81c). Autoimmune enteropathy, giardiasis and cow's

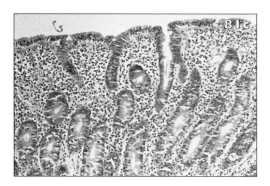

milk-sensitive enteropathy may also cause a flat mucosa. If villous atrophy is demonstrated, the child is placed on a strict gluten-free diet.

74

82 A 29-year-old nurse was investigated for a 12-month history of problematic watery diarrhoea. On examination she was thin (body mass index 18.5 kg/m²) but otherwise well with no abdominal or sigmoidoscopic signs. Investigations revealed normal full blood count; renal, hepatic and thyroid biochemistry, ESR and CRP within the normal range; and several normal microbiological examinations of the stool. The average daily stool weight was 650 g during 3 days' in-patient observation, with an average of 5.2 g fat per day. Rectal biopsy was normal, as was a barium follow-through study. The stool osmolality was 235 mosmol/kg, and alkalinization of the urine with sodium hydroxide produced a pink colour.
i. What is the diagnosis?
ii. How can this be confirmed?

83 A 32-year-old woman with a background history of recurrent abdominal pain for 16 years presents to the emergency room with a 4-day history of diffuse abdominal pain, cramping in nature and worse in both lower quadrants. The pain is associated with vomiting, constipation, a low-grade fever and weakness. She has a rash on her hands which she believes is related to her anxiety episodes and 'allergies' as it is worse in the summer months and when she is outdoors. She also reports that her skin is unduly fragile. She has been admitted to several area hospitals for the pain, which has required narcotic analgesics and may take up to a week to settle. She has major depression and has undergone numerous abdomino-pelvic surgeries which have not impacted on her pain episodes. Extensive radiological and endoscopic examinations failed to identify a structural abnormality. She takes omeprazole and methadone. She has a daughter with irritable bowel and psychiatric symptoms. Examination revealed facial hypertrichosis, blistering and scarring of her hands (83), a soft abdomen with diffuse tenderness but normal bowel sounds, and symmetric limb weakness. Blood pressure is normal and pulse 108/min. Blood count, BUN and serum amylase are normal. Serum sodium is 126 mmol/l and potassium is normal. There are no cells in the urine which is dark and tests negative for blood.
i. Discuss the diagnostic possibilities.
ii. What is the likely diagnosis, and comment on the clinical features.
iii. Discuss the pathophysiology of this disorder.
iv. How may the diagnosis be confirmed?
v. Discuss treatment of this patient.

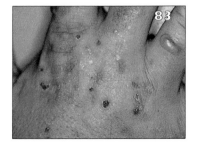

82 & 83: Answers

82 i. Differential diagnosis includes microscopic colitis since rectal biopsy without more proximal colonic histology may be misleading. Coeliac disease also remains a possibility. However, the pink colour change when the urine is alkalinized is almost diagnostic; it is highly suggestive of the presence of phenolphthalein, a common constituent of over-the-counter laxatives. The likely diagnosis is laxative abuse.
ii. The stool osmolality helps to identify patients who dilute the stool with urine or tap water. Normally the stool osmolality equates to that of the plasma (280–295 mosmol/kg) since the colon does not secrete free water. If the stool osmolality is substantially low, dilution is confirmed. Measurement of urea or creatinine in the stool reveals whether urine is the contaminant.

Laxative abuse is confirmed by high-performance thin-layer liquid chromatography of the urine, which detects anthraquinolones (senna, cascara, etc.), bisacodyl and phenolphthalein. It may be necessary to perform estimations on several occasions if laxative use is episodic.

83 i. This patient has recurrent severe abdominal pain for which no structural cause has been identified. Possibilities include irritable bowel syndrome and a psychiatric disorder. However, in view of the possible systemic features and low serum sodium, connective tissue disease (e.g. SLE and polyarteritis nodosum), heavy-metal toxicity, endocrine disorders, sarcoidosis, syphilis and amyloidosis need to be considered.
ii. The combination of neuropsychiatric and dermatological manifestations, with the family history suggests porphyria [variegate or hereditary coproporphyria (HCP)]. Neurological symptoms may sometimes mimic Guillain–Barré syndrome, and severe hyponatraemia due to SIADH may occur.
iii. Porphyria results from inherited enzyme disorders of the haem biosynthetic pathway. Specific enzyme deficiencies along this pathway lead to an accumulation of excessive porphyrins and/or porphyrin precursors – and specific syndromes. Defects early in the pathway cause excess porphobilinogen (PBG) and delta-aminolaevulinic acid (ALA), which cause neurological manifestations. Psychiatric manifestations are common, and seizures may occur. Accumulation of distal pathway substrates (uroporphyrins, coproporphyrins and protoporphyrins) cause cutaneous manifestations. Both are seen in variegate porphyria (VP).
iv. Diagnosis of acute neuroporphyria may be confirmed by urine PBG and ALA. Auto-oxidation of PBG causes the urine to darken on standing. In VP and HCP the urine may be negative during remission, but stool protoporphyrin or coproporphyrin III are elevated.
v. Treatment consists of adequate intake of fluid and carbohydrates and avoidance of porphyrinogenic medications (e.g. barbiturates, sulphonamides, steroids, alcohol). Serum sodium is monitored. Opiates and phenothiazines are safe for pain control and for agitation and psychosis, respectively. Beta-blockers are useful for tachycardia and hypertension, and diazepam is safe if seizures occur. Use of haematin is controversial. Oral contraceptives help symptoms related to the menstrual cycle. Family screening and counselling are important.

84 Match each of the following statements (i–v) concerning screening for colorectal carcinoma with the appropriate percentage range (a–e).
i. Decrease in incidence of colorectal carcinoma following prior colonoscopic removal of all colonic polyps.
ii. Reduction in mortality from colorectal carcinoma as a result of annual faecal occult blood testing.
iii. Decrease in mortality from colorectal carcinoma as a result of screening sigmoidoscopy. (The decrease is for lesions within reach of the instrument.)
iv. Percentage of screening faecal occult blood tests (non-hydrated) that are positive.
v. Positive predictive value (for colorectal carcinoma) of a positive screening faecal occult blood test.
a. 2–4%
b. 10%
c. 25–33%
d. 59–80%
e. 76–90%

85 A 66-year-old woman with NSAID-dependent rheumatoid arthritis presented with dyspepsia and weight loss of 3.5 kg (8 lb) over 3 months. She attributed the latter to anorexia since her symptoms were exacerbated by ingestion of food. Upper GI series revealed an ulcer on the high lesser curve of the stomach. She was treated with an 8-week course of omeprazole for a presumed NSAID-associated ulcer and was scheduled for an upper endoscopy 6 weeks later for biopsies and to document ulcer healing. Because of her severe arthritis, NSAIDs were continued throughout the treatment period. At endoscopy, a persistent ulcer was found (85a) and biopsied (85b). A rapid urease test for *Helicobacter pylori*, performed on an antral biopsy specimen obtained endoscopically, is positive.

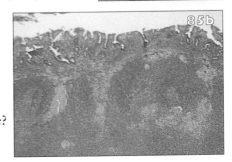

i. Should patients with gastric ulcers undergo follow-up endoscopy?
ii. Must the patient discontinue NSAIDs in addition to receiving antisecretory therapy?
iii. What causes of ulcers other than NSAIDs are sought in this situation?
iv. What treatment should she receive?

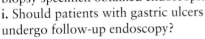

84 i. (e) Results from the National Polyp Study in the US demonstrate a significant decrease in the incidence in colorectal carcinoma following prior removal of all colon adenomas.
ii. (c) Randomized, prospective and case-controlled studies have demonstrated a favourable impact on colorectal mortality from annual screening by faecal occult-blood testing.
iii. (d) Case-control studies have shown that screening with flexible sigmoidoscopy has the potential to reduce both the incidence and mortality of cancer.
iv. (a) Less than 5% of those screened have a positive faecal occult blood test. Hydration of slides , however, produces a four-fold increase in positive tests, including many false-positives – and a high rate of colonoscopy.
v. (b) Approximately one-third of asymptomatic patients aged over 50 years who undergo screening with stool occult blood testing will harbour a neoplastic lesion. Two-thirds of these are benign lesions. Polyps responsible for positive tests are usually greater than 1.5 cm in diameter. Discovery of smaller lesions is considered serendipitous.

85 i. Patients taking NSAIDS are at risk for ulcer disease. The presence of *Helicobacter pylori* (HP) gastritis may constitute an additional risk factor, and both need to be addressed from a therapeutic point of view. Classic teaching holds that all patients with gastric ulcers require documentation of complete healing either endoscopically or radiologically. This also serves to confirm the ulcer's benign nature. The cost-effectiveness of this strategy has recently been questioned.
ii. Every effort is made to discontinue NSAID therapy while the ulcer is treated. Unfortunately, this is not always possible, and NSAID administration may need to be continued because of severely symptomatic arthritis. Such patients may benefit from the addition of misoprostol for ulcer prophylaxis after the index ulcer has healed.
iii. Factors associated with poor healing include an underlying malignancy, non-compliance with medications, and continuing NSAID use. In this case, HP gastritis was tested for at the time of endoscopy using a rapid urease test. While a positive test confirms the presence of the organism, a negative test may be misleading in the presence of proton pump inhibition which may suppress but not eradicate the infection. HP infection itself is commonly associated with a marked lymphocytic response in the gastric mucosa, which may mimic a 'pseudolymphoma'. Occasionally, this lymphocytic response becomes autonomous, leading to the clonal expansion of a specific precursor cell and a true low-grade lymphoma. This patient had a non-healing ulcer due to a MALToma. The histology (**85b**) demonstrates sheets of small lymphocytes, which are relatively indolent low-grade lymphomas localized to the gastric wall. Imaging, and occasionally laparotomy, may be necessary to exclude more extensive disease.
iv. Virtually all gastric MALTomas are associated with HP gastritis, and up to 50% resolve with antibiotic treatment alone. An oncology consultation is sought.

86 A 14-year-old boy from Malta presented with a 2-year history of abdominal discomfort, exaggerated bowel sounds and loose stools. He thought there was a link with milk ingestion. On examination he was well apart from being obese, with a weight above the 97th centile. Among investigations seeking an explanation for his symptoms he underwent a lactose hydrogen breath test (86).

Discuss the result and its diagnostic significance.

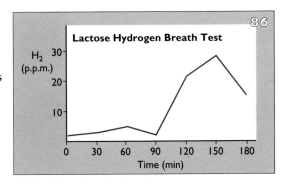

87 The biopsies 87a and 87b are from adult patients whose only symptoms were chronic diarrhoea with minimal weight loss. Physical examination, colonoscopy and upper endoscopy are unremarkable in both.
i. What is the diagnosis in each patient?
ii. Describe stool abnormalities that may be present in each disorder.
iii. Comment on other possible gastrointestinal involvement in each disorder.
iv. Describe disorders associated with each diagnosis.
v. Discuss treatment of each patient.

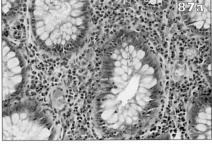

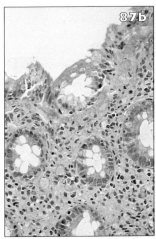

86 Normally, there are only traces of hydrogen in expired air. If carbohydrate is not absorbed in the small intestine it is fermented by colonic bacteria and produces hydrogen which is absorbed and excreted in larger quantities than normal via the lungs. The peak is seen 1–3 hours after carbohydrate ingestion, when the unabsorbed sugar reaches the colon. The use of lactose in the test and the obviously positive result demonstrated (normal is <20 p.p.m. or an increase of <10 p.p.m. above baseline) indicate malabsorption. Rapid transit or small bowel bacterial overgrowth can produce a similar picture. Equally, the demonstration of lactose malabsorption does not yield a diagnosis of alactasia or lactose intolerance unless other less selective causes of its malabsorption are excluded. The occurrence of typical symptoms during the test are helpful pointers. The patient described had no other abnormal investigations and did well on a lactose-free diet supervised by a dietician. Avoidance of overt dietary lactose is usually sufficient to achieve control, and traces of 'hidden' lactose in foods that are not obviously milk-based do not usually pose problems.

87 i. 87a demonstrates eosinophilic infiltration of the mucosa, consistent with eosinophilic colitis. 87b shows a subepithelial layer of dense collagen, diagnostic of collagenous colitis.
ii. Stools may be normal in the former, but a protein-losing enteropathy or steatorrhoea may occur. Charcot–Leyden crystals due to extrusion of eosinophils may be seen. Parasites may be present. In collagenous colitis the stools are watery, and decrease with fasting.
iii. Eosinophilic gastroenteritis (EGE) may involve the mucosa (mucosal thickening, ulceration, masses, malabsorption), muscularis (obstructive symptoms), or serosa (ascites). Biliary, hepatic or pancreatic involvement rarely occurs. Collagenous colitis may be prevalent more proximally. Rectal biopsy is therefore not a sensitive screen. The small bowel may also be involved.
iv. Food hypersensitivity is found in children with EGE. About half are atopic. The differential diagnosis includes hypereosinophilia syndrome, parasitic infestation and periarteritis nodosa. Eosinophilic granuloma is characterized by intramural collections of eosinophils producing a mass, often gastric in location. Collagenous colitis is predominantly a disease of females and is associated with arthritis, autoimmune disorders and coeliac disease. Non-steroidal anti-inflammatory drugs may play a role.
v. Dietary manipulation has been disappointing in EGE. Conventional antidiarrhoeals may be sufficient for mild cases. Most cases respond to prednisone. Disodium cromoglycate may be useful. Mild cases of collagenous colitis respond to antidiarrhoeal medications. 5-ASA may be used for non-responders. Steroids are used for intractable cases.

88 The lesion shown (88) was found in the descending colon of a 45-year-old man attending for colonoscopic follow-up after a right hemicolectomy for a caecal carcinoma.
i. Describe the endoscopic findings (88), and speculate on the likely histology.
ii. Discuss the molecular biology of this lesion.
iii. How should this patient be managed?

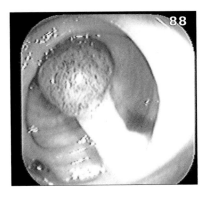

89 A 32-year-old man – a life-long heavy drinker – had been admitted several times with acute abdominal pain over the 12 months that preceded the admission during which this CT scan was taken (89).
i. What does the CT scan show?
ii. Of what symptoms may the patient complain?
iii. How should this patient be managed?

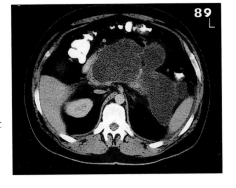

90 A 47-year-old man complained of 4 years of recurrent heartburn and water brash. He also had a 3-month history of intermittent dysphagia, but no weight loss.
i. What does the endoscopy picture in 90 show?
ii. What is the aetiology of this condition?
iii. How would you treat this condition?
iv. Are there any complications of this condition?

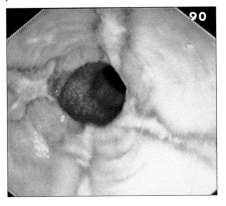

88–90: Answers

88 i. A pedunculated polyp projects into the colonic lumen, which is most likely to be an adenoma. Some 75% of colorectal adenomas are of tubular architecture, 10% are villous, and 15% are tubulovillous on histology. The larger the polyp, the greater the chance of dysplasia or invasive carcinoma.
ii. A complex series of mutations is thought to result in the adenoma–carcinoma sequence. The *APC*, *p53* and *MCC* genes are important tumour-suppressor genes, whereas *k-ras* and *c-myc* are probably the most relevant oncogenes in colonic neoplasia.
iii. The polyp should be removed by diathermy snare and if confirmed as a benign adenoma, further interval colonic surveillance is necessary.

89 i. Multiple pancreatic pseudocysts. Collections of pancreatic fluid and liquefied tissue, they form in the pancreatic or peripancreatic tissues. Their walls comprise granulation and fibrous tissue, with no epithelial lining (hence, pseudocyst).
ii. Abdominal pain, steatorrhoea, or diabetes. Pseudocysts may indent the stomach and cause vomiting or distort the common bile duct, inducing biliary stasis.
iii. Pseudocysts <10 cm in diameter often resolve spontaneously. If no improvement has occurred after 6 weeks, intervention should be considered. Without drainage, large pseudocysts may rupture or cause massive haemorrhage. Drainage can be performed surgically, percutaneously or by interventional endoscopy.

90 i. Moderate oesophagitis.
ii. The LOS forms the main barrier to reflux of gastric contents into the oesophagus; the majority of reflux episodes occur during its spontaneous relaxation. In oesophagitis, reflux episodes occur more frequently and the normal suppression of reflux when supine or asleep is lost. In severe oesophagitis, further free gastro-oesophageal reflux occurs. A hiatus hernia predisposes to gastro-oesophageal reflux.
iii. The mainstay of medical treatment is acid suppression therapy. Mild reflux symptoms can often be relieved with antacids, but some patients require proton pump inhibitors. Following healing and cessation of treatment, relapse is frequent. Surgery may also be considered. The most favoured operation is a Nissen fundoplication (now developed as a laparoscopic procedure) intended to prevent reflux by wrapping the fundus around the distal oesophagus.
iv. Bleeding, oesophageal stricture and, probably, Barrett's oesophagus.

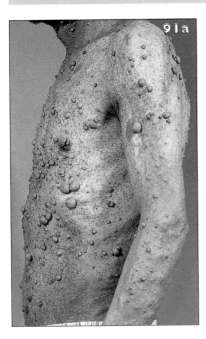

91 i. Describe the abnormalities seen in 91a and 91b.
ii. What are the respective diagnoses?
iii. How is each inherited?
iv. Discuss how each disorder may affect the gastrointestinal tract.
v. Are these disorders associated with gastrointestinal malignancies?

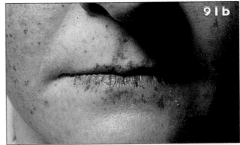

92 Colonoscopy was performed in a 56-year-old man with a 25-year history of rectal bleeding that he had attributed to haemorrhoids. The appearances in the distal colon (92a) and in the proximal ascending colon (92b) are shown.
i. What is the underlying diagnosis?
ii. What else has happened?
iii. What measures should be taken to avoid this?
iv. What is the correct management for this man now?

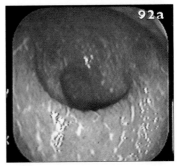

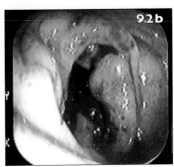

91 & 92: Answers

91 i. Multiple neurofibromas. Other cutaneous lesions include *café au lait* macules and axillary freckles. Mucocutaneous pigmentation is present in the patient in **91b** (darker than conventional freckles and crossing the vermilion border).
ii. Neurofibromatosis (Von Recklinghausen's disease) and Peutz–Jeghers syndrome.
iii. Neurofibromatosis is an autosomal dominant disorder affecting 1 in 3000–4000 persons. The NF1 gene has been localized to chromosome 17q. Peutz–Jeghers syndrome is also inherited via an autosomal dominant mechanism. The degree of penetrance is high.
iv. Neurofibromatosis types NF1 and NF3 (familial intestinal neurofibromatosis) may affect the gastrointestinal tract where luminal lesions may be silent, or may ulcerate, bleed, be responsible for obstruction, intussusception or perforation. They are generally submucosal and multiple. Gastroparesis and intestinal and colonic dysmotility (including pseudo-obstruction and megacolon) may also occur. Gastrointestinal leiomyomas, sarcomas and other neurogenic neoplasms have also been reported. Gastrointestinal hamartomatous polyps occur in over 90% of patients with Peutz–Jeghers syndrome, over two-thirds in the small intestine, but also in the colon and stomach. Larger polyps may infarct, ulcerate, bleed and lead to intussusception. Symptoms generally appear after age 10 years.
v. Sarcomatous transformation of neurofibromas may occur. Ileal adenocarcinomas with concurrent leiomyomas have been reported. Up to 13% of patients with Peutz–Jeghers syndrome develop gastrointestinal carcinomas, especially in the stomach and duodenum. The risk of colon cancer is substantially lower than in adenomatosis polyposis, but it is prudent to survey patients whose colonic hamartomatous polyps contain adenomatous elements. Numerous extra-intestinal tumours also occur, elevating the lifetime risk of malignancy to around 50%.

92 i. Ulcerative colitis. Findings include prominent tortuous vessels, petechiae formation on minimal instrumental trauma, opaque granular mucosa, and patchy erythema. As the disease becomes more severe, the inflamed mucosa may become covered with a purulent exudate, 'bear-claw ulcers' may develop, and there may be free blood and mucus in the lumen.
ii. Colonic carcinoma complicating ulcerative colitis. Ulcerative colitis poses an overall 11-fold increase in the risk of colorectal cancer. This is related to the extent of the disease. Patients with proctitis or rectosigmoiditis are at relatively little risk, while the risk in extensive colitis is around 10% by 20 years of disease.
iii. Patients with long-standing extensive colitis should probably undergo regular surveillance by colonoscopy and multiple biopsy, perhaps at 2-year intervals after 10 years. Dysplasia is usually an indication for colectomy.
iv. The patient requires a total colectomy with either formation of an ileostomy or a pouch construction. Any less radical surgery allows the possibility of development of further lesions in the remaining affected bowel.

93 Match the following (i–v) with the appropriate function (a–e) concerning vitamin B_{12} absorption:
i. R-protein.
ii. Intrinsic factor.
iii. Gastric acid.
iv. Ileal receptor.
v. Hepatic secretion.
a. Liberates dietary methyl cobalamin from ingested food.
b. Production stimulated by cyclic-AMP agonists.
c. Degraded by pancreatic proteases.
d. Disposes of inactive cobalamin in serum.
e. Located in pits between adjacent brush-border villi.

94 Two young men both present with dysphagia and undergo upper gastrointestinal endoscopy. The first patient complains of intermittent dysphagia for solids. No weight loss or systemic complaints have occurred. He has undergone a prior barium examination (94a). The finding at endoscopy is shown in 94b. The second patient is known to have AIDS and complains of persistent low retrosternal pain, and dysphagia for liquids and solids. He is afraid to eat and has lost a considerable amount of weight. His endoscopy (94c) demonstrates a large discrete ulcer in the distal oesophagus. Biopsies and cultures are negative for pathogens. There is no evidence for gastro-oesophageal reflux. For each patient:

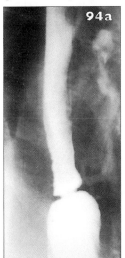

i. What is the diagnosis?
ii. What is the pathogenesis of the lesion?
iii. How do they commonly present?
iv. Comment on management.
v. What is the prognosis for recurrence?

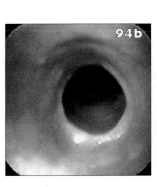

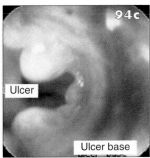

93 i. (c)
ii. (b)
iii. (a)
iv. (e)
v. (d)
Gastric acid liberates dietary methyl cobalamin from ingested food which binds preferentially to endogenous R proteins of salivary origin. Intrinsic factor, like acid, a product of the parietal cell, has less affinity for cobalamin in an acid environment, but readily binds to free biologically active cobalamin in the small intestine once the salivary R protein (bound to cobalamin in the stomach) is degraded by pancreatic proteases. Cobalamin analogues of bacterial origin with even minor structural changes do not bind to intrinsic factor. The intrinsic factor–cobalamin complex undergoes a conformational change that renders the complex resistant to proteolysis. This complex binds to the ileal receptor located in pits between adjacent brush-border ileal villi in a highly specific, rapid and energy-independent process. Transcobalamin II, a cobalamin-binding protein, delivers cobalamin to body tissues. Transcobalamin III, a plasma R protein, binds excess cobalamin and inactive cobalamin analogues for hepatic uptake and secretion into bile. Disorders affecting acid production, parietal cell function, proximal small intestine, pancreatic enzyme generation and function, and ileal disorders, may potentially interfere with vitamin B_{12} absorption. Furthermore, certain bacteria compete for uptake of luminal cobalamin, even if bound to intrinsic factor. Some drugs (e.g. biguanides, p-aminosalicylate) interfere with ileal uptake of cobalamin.

94 i. The first patient has a Schatski (distal oesophageal mucosal, or B-) ring, and the patient with AIDS has an idiopathic oesophageal ulcer.
ii. The Schatski ring is a mucosal ring at the squamocolumnar junction, generally considered to represent a congenital structural variant, but gastro-oesophageal reflux may be an aggravating factor. The 'idiopathic' oesophageal ulcer may only be diagnosed once opportunistic infection or pill-oesophagitis is excluded. Occasionally, a neoplasm presents as an ulcerated lesion.
iii. Patients with Schatski rings are generally asymptomatic until the intraluminal diameter becomes less than 13 mm. Intermittent dysphagia for solids is then classic, including the 'steakhouse syndrome'. AIDS patients with an idiopathic oesophageal ulcer generally present with lower substernal pain, odynophagia and unremitting dysphagia. Occasionally, a gastrointestinal bleed is the first indication.
iv. The symptomatic Schatski ring requires dilatation – generally at the time of endoscopic diagnosis. The ring is torn and luminal patency re-established. Corticosteroid therapy (oral or intralesional) is considered for idiopathic oesophageal ulcer. Acid reduction and thalidomide may also help.
v. The majority of patients have no further swallowing difficulty after initial treatment of the Schatski ring. However, repeat dilatation may be necessary in those with thicker rings and gastro-oesophageal reflux. The majority of patients with an idiopathic oesophageal ulcer respond to corticosteroid therapy, but larger lesions may take many months to re-epithelialize. Repeat sampling after a few weeks or if symptoms prove intractable is important to ensure that an opportunistic infection is not present.

95 A 32-year-old HIV-positive man
presents with fever, weight loss,
abdominal pain, and diarrhoea. The
CD4+ lymphocyte count is 150/ml
(normal, >500/ml). An upper GI series
with small-bowel follow-through shows
thickened mucosal folds from the distal
duodenum and proximal small bowel to
the mid-ileum suggestive of Whipple's

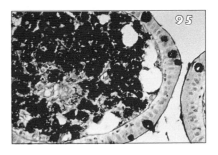

disease. Mucosal biopsies of the
abnormal-appearing bowel are stained with PAS (95).
i. Should any other special stains be performed?
ii. Does this patient have Whipple's disease?
iii. What other areas of the body are likely to be involved?
iv. Should imaging studies be performed to identify other involved organs?
v. How should he be treated?

96 A 35-year-old man with a history of recurrent upper respiratory tract
infections, bipolar disorder since the age of 18 years, hypothyroidism, mild
mental retardation since birth and obesity, presents to the emergency room
with vomiting and regurgitation of food, particularly when bending forward.
Three months previously he underwent an upper endoscopy after a
haematemesis which revealed grade 3–4 severe oesophagitis. He was placed
on H2 receptor antagonists. Because of persistent heartburn, vomiting and a
lack of improvement, he was switched to omeprazole. A repeat upper
endoscopy (96a) is performed and a 24-hour ambulatory oesophageal pH
study (96b) obtained.
i. What is the likely diagnosis?
ii. Comment on the endoscopic appearance in 96a.
iii. What additional medical measures may be
appropriate?
iv. Comment on the study demonstrated in 96b.
v. What else may be done should these steps fail?

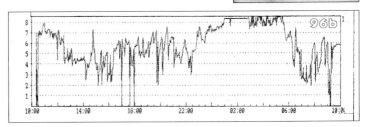

95 i. Whipple's disease, as well as infection caused by *Mycobacterium avium* complex (MAC), is characterized by the presence of PAS-positive foamy macrophages in the lamina propria. MAC (pseudo-Whipple's) is commonly seen in late-stage AIDS. The macrophages contain numerous acid-fast bacilli (the Whipple's bacillus itself is not acid-fast). Thus, an acid-fast stain may be used to distinguish readily between the two disorders (**95**).
ii. The clinical setting suggests MAC infection.
iii. MAC commonly disseminates to other areas of the body in HIV patients including the bone marrow, lymph nodes, stomach, large bowel, liver and lung. Blood cultures may be positive. In patients with AIDS, intestinal TB is also a possibility. However, PAS-positive macrophages are not seen here.
iv. CT scan of the abdomen would probably reveal adenopathy, and possibly enlargement of the liver and spleen. Little is to be gained clinically by identifying other areas of involvement in the absence of symptoms, so these studies are not clinically indicated.
v. MAC infections are extremely difficult to treat and therapy is suboptimal. Current therapy in AIDS patients consists of maintenance multi-drug regimens containing rifampcin, ethambutol, amikacin and/or ciprofloxacin.

96 i. Gastro-oesophageal reflux disease (GORD). Persistent symptoms in spite of anti-secretory therapy suggests progressive disease or complications. Dysphagia, nocturnal pain, regurgitation of food and weight loss are alarm symptoms. Further evaluation includes barium oesophagogram or preferably endoscopy. No evidence for severe mucosal disease or a stricture suggests motor dysfunction, which is confirmed using oesophageal manometry. The degree of acid reflux may be quantified by a 24-hour pH study.
ii. This endoscopic view (**96a**) of the lower third of the oesophagus demonstrates erythema and erosions, but there are no large ulcers, scars or strictures. A hiatal hernia may also be seen.
iii. Weight reduction, raising the head of the bed, and avoiding restrictive clothing relieves symptoms in up to 60% of individuals with GORD. Vigorous acid suppression with high-dose H2 receptor antagonists or proton pump blockers may be necessary. The addition of a prokinetic agent (e.g. cisapride) before meals and at night may alleviate the vomiting, and promotes oesophageal peristalsis and gastric emptying.
iv. 96b is a 24-hour pH profile. The pH sensor is placed 5 cm (2 in) above the lower oesophageal sphincter and a continuous recording obtained. This study demonstrates severe postprandial acid reflux with pH dropping below 4.0; the oesophageal pH was below 4 for 7% of the time (normal: <4.5%). This indicates that the patient has significant acid reflux, particularly after meals. Manometry showed poor oesophageal peristalsis and reduced lower oesophageal sphincter tone.
v. Surgery is considered when symptoms persist despite medical therapy. Fundoplication may now be performed laparoscopically.

97 Match each of the following antidiarrhoeal therapies (i–v) with the statement (a–e) that best describes its mechanism of action:
i. Opiates.
ii. Alpha-2-adrenergic agonists.
iii. Octreotide.
iv. Corticosteroids.
v. Oral rehydration fluids.
a. Activate(s) the sodium-dependent co-transport by the presence of luminal solutes such as glucose and certain amino acids.
b. Stimulate(s) electroneutral sodium chloride absorption and inhibition of anion secretion.
c. Convert(s) propulsive contractions to segmental contractions, thereby prolonging transit and increasing efficiency of absorption.
d. Increase(s) the number of sodium channels in the luminal membrane of the distal colon to increase electrogenic sodium absorption.
e. Inhibit(s) hormone secretion produced by endocrine tumours.

98 A 33-year-old woman with AIDS presents with a 5-week history of abdominal pain, diarrhoea and rectal bleeding, intermittent fevers and 7 kg (15 lb) weight loss. The diarrhoea is profuse, up to 10 times during the day, and wakes her from sleep. She has a history of *Candida* oesophagitis, *Pneumocystis carinii* pneumonitis and cytomegalovirus retinitis. Her most recent CD4+ count was 24/mm^3. She is afebrile with a soft but diffusely tender abdomen. An anal ulcer is present. Haemoglobin is 10.9 g/dl, WBC cell count 2.9×10^9/l (2900/mm^3) and serum electrolytes are normal. Faecal leukocyte stain is positive. Routine stool cultures, *C. difficile* toxin and ova and parasite examinations are negative. The response to antidiarrhoeals is suboptimal. Abdominal radiography suggests oedematous colonic mucosa and colonoscopy demonstrates patchy erythema and ulceration throughout the colon (98a). Biopsies are performed (98b).

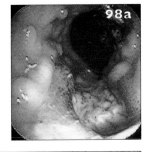

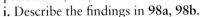

i. Describe the findings in 98a, 98b.
ii. What is the diagnosis?
iii. Are confirmatory tests necessary?
iv. Discuss the pathogenesis and complications of this disorder.
v. Describe treatment of this condition.

97 i. (c) Opiates affect intestinal motility by reducing propulsive motor and increasing segmental smooth muscle contractions. This prolongs transit time and increases contact time between the absorptive surface and luminal fluid, increasing absorption and reducing diarrhoea. Opiates may also suppress the activities of secretomotor neurones on intestinal electrolyte transport.

ii. (b) Alpha-2-adrenergic agonists are useful in diabetic diarrhoea, correcting alpha-adrenergic-derived regulation of intestinal fluid and electrolyte transport by stimulating electroneutral sodium chloride absorption and inhibiting anion secretion in the enterocyte plasma membrane. Inhibition of enteric nerve-stimulated and centrally mediated secretion and smooth muscle effects may also be important.

iii. (e) Octreotide decreases propulsive and increases segmental contractions. It increases absorption and decreases secretion of water and electrolytes through direct actions on enterocytes and indirectly through neural and other lamina propria cells. It also inhibits secretion of endocrine tumours that cause diarrhoea, such as VIPomas and carcinoids.

iv. (d) Steroids reduce diarrhoea by stimulating electroneutral sodium chloride absorption, increasing electrogenic sodium absorption in the colon, possibly by increasing the expression of additional sodium channels, and by increasing $Na^+-K^+-ATPase$ activity. The last effect is seen over several days. They also inhibit inflammatory mediators responsible for the diarrhoea of inflammatory bowel disease.

v. (a) Oral rehydration solutions promote absorption, but do not affect the secretory process. Monosaccharides such as glucose stimulate fluid and electrolyte absorption by promoting a solvent drag effect and activate the sodium-dependent glucose co-transporter. Their active transport promotes sodium and water absorption. Although diarrhoeal volume may increase, metabolic imbalances are rapidly corrected.

98 i. There are discrete deep ulcers present throughout the colon. Intranuclear inclusions of CMV are present.

ii. CMV colitis. GI involvement is the second most common focus after eye disease.

iii. Immunoperoxidase staining for CMV is usually positive in this situation. No further diagnostic testing is necessary before beginning antiviral therapy. Circulating CMV-infected endothelial cells may be detected in cytospin preparations of peripheral blood cells by immunoperoxidase staining for CMV intermediate antigen – and correlate with active infection.

iv. Up to 50% of patients with advanced HIV infection have reactivated CMV in blood leukocytes. CMV commonly infects endothelial cells, induces localized procoagulant activity, and causes adherence of neutrophils to endothelial cells. Infection induces vasculitis, which in turn results in thrombosis leading to ischaemia, necrosis and ulceration. CMV infection typically occurs late in the course of AIDS when the CD4+ lymphocyte count is $<150/mm^3$. CMV infection is the most common cause of acute lower GI haemorrhage, megacolon and bowel perforation in patients with AIDS.

v. Ganciclovir is generally used. The optimal duration of treatment is unknown and recrudescence of infection may occur following its withdrawal. Viral resistance to ganciclovir increases with duration of therapy. Foscarnet, a virostatic agent, has also proved useful. Unremitting colitis may require surgery.

99 A 49-year-old patient on dialysis for chronic renal failure due to SLE has experienced upper abdominal discomfort after meals for several months. It has been refractory to H2-receptor antagonists and omeprazole. No loss of appetite, weight change, vomiting or change in bowel habit has occurred. Physical examination reveals her to be mildly cushingoid, but apart from some tenderness in the epigastrium, her presentation is unremarkable. The renal profile is stable and the liver enzymes are normal. An upper gastrointestinal endoscopy revealed a nodular duodenum (99a).

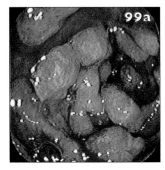

i. Discuss the differential diagnosis.
ii. What additional investigations are appropriate?
iii. Comment on the endoscopic findings.
iv. What additional work-up/manoeuvre may be necessary?
v. Discuss management strategy.

100 A new-born infant has bilious vomiting after initial feedings. The 34-week pregnancy was complicated by polyhydramnios. The infant (100a) is noted to be slightly cyanotic, generally hypotonic with a flat occiput and small head. Simian lines are on both palms and a single flexion crease is on the fifth finger. A 3/6 pansystolic cardiac murmur is heard. An abdominal radiograph is performed (100b).

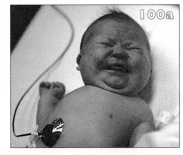

i. What diagnosis do the morphological features suggest?
ii. Describe the radiological features, and the likely intra-abdominal abnormality.
iii. Describe how this disorder may present.
iv. How is this entity best diagnosed and treated?
v. Which associated disorders are considered?

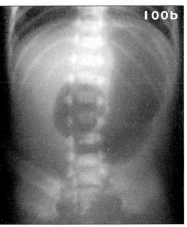

99 & 100: Answers

99 i. Peptic ulcer disease, GORD or oesophagitis. Renal impairment also leads to pancreatitis. The vasculitis and serositis that accompany SLE may cause a peritonitis syndrome, gut ischaemia or acalculous cholecystitis.

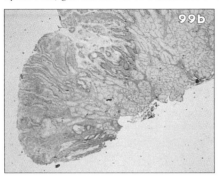

ii. Endoscopy, ultrasonography and CT scanning; serum amylase and lipase are unreliable tests of pancreatic disease in renal impairment.
iii. A nodular duodenitis from Brunner's gland hyperplasia.
iv. The abnormal mucosa should be biopsied; hypertrophied Brunner's glands and inflammation are typical (99b).
v. As these lesions rarely cause symptoms, an alternative origin for symptoms should be considered.

100 i. Trisomy 21, or Down syndrome.
ii. The 'double-bubble' of duodenal stenosis or atresia, with a gas-filled and dilated stomach and a gas-filled dilated duodenum.
iii. Duodenal atresia occurs in 1 per 10000 live births, comprising almost 50% of all cases of intestinal atresia. It may involve the region distal (20%) or proximal (80%) to the ampulla of Vater, leading to bilious or non-bilious vomiting usually of the first day of life. It is pressaged by polyhydramnios in 40% of cases and prematurity in 50%.
iv. Diagnosis consists of upper gastrointestinal contrast studies (100c). Treatment consists of duodenojejunostomy (100d).
v. Congenital cardiac lesion (30–50% of children with Trisomy 21).

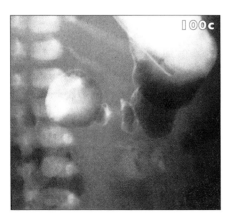

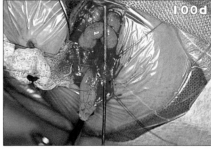

101 A previously healthy 2-year-old child presents with massive haematochezia. Physical examination reveals an alert but pale child with a heart rate of 160/min and blood pressure of 90/45 mmHg. Her abdomen is non-tender with no palpable mass. Rectal examination is normal. The abdominal radiograph is normal.
i. Discuss initial management.
ii. What diagnosis is most likely?
iii. Describe its embryology.
iv. How may the diagnosis be confirmed?
v. Discuss further management.

102 An 87-year-old man had a palliative procedure (**102a**) for his carcinoma of the oesophagus.
i. What is the procedure in **102a**?
ii. What are the indications for this procedure?
iii. What complication is shown by the second radiograph (**102b**)?
iv. How might the patient have presented with this complication?
v. What other complications occur following this procedure?

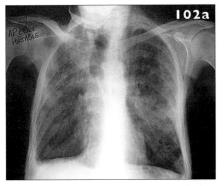

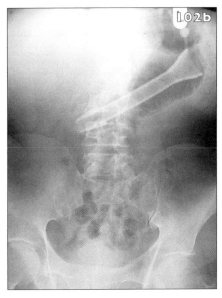

101 i. It is essential to assure haemodynamic stability. A large-bore catheter is inserted and blood obtained for cross-matching. Lower gastrointestinal bleeding in a child may be caused by a rapidly bleeding source in the upper gastrointestinal tract. Therefore, a gastric lavage is performed.

ii. Massive painless haematochezia is most consistent with bleeding from a Meckel's diverticulum.

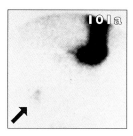

iii. Meckel's diverticulum is a vestige of the vitelline duct which connects the midgut to the yolk sac. At 5–7 weeks, the duct normally obliterates. In 2% of cases, the intestinal end of the duct remains, leaving a diverticulum on the antimesenteric border of the ileum, approximately 80 cm from the ileocaecal valve. About 50% of these structures contain ectopic gastric mucosa which secretes acid, causing ulceration and bleeding.

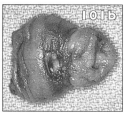

iv. ^{99m}Tc pertechnetate nuclear scan (Meckel's scan) can demonstrate ectopic gastric mucosa in the right lower quadrant (101a, arrow). The sensitivity of this study is about 75% but improves to 90% if H2 blockers are administered for 24 hours before testing.

v. Surgical removal is the definitive treatment for a Meckel's diverticulum that has bled (101b). If the scan is negative, however, colonoscopy must be considered before exploration to rule out other causes of haematochezia.

102 i. An Atkinson tube has been placed across the tumour to maintain a patent oesophageal lumen.

ii. Indications include:
• Inoperable oesophageal cancer and dysphagia.
• Extrinsic pressure on the oesophagus, usually by mediastinal or lung malignancy.
• To seal a perforation of tracheo-oesophageal fistula due to malignant disease.
The use of Atkinson tubes in the treatment of benign oesophageal disease is controversial.

iii. The tube has slipped from position and is lying in the stomach.

iv. The patient probably developed a recurrence of dysphagia. He may also have developed abdominal pain if the tube caused upper gastrointestinal tract obstruction or perforation.

v. Apart from the tube slipping from position, it is not uncommon for oesophageal perforations to occur during insertion of the tube. These can usually be sealed with the tube itself. Bleeding may occur, particularly if there is reflux oesophagitis secondary to loss of competency of the lower oesophageal sphincter. Aspiration of gastric contents may also occur for the same reason. Perforation of the stomach is less easy to resolve and mortality is high. Recurrence of dysphagia due to bolus obstruction or recurrent tumour is not uncommon. Tumour overgrowth can be treated by injection with alcohol or Nd:YAG laser therapy.

103 A 14-year-old girl with a life-long
tendency to loose stools presented with
discomfort in the right hypochondrium
and itching. Apart from localized
tenderness, examination was normal.
Investigations demonstrated abnormal
liver function tests with a predominantly
hepatic picture and a bilirubin level three
times the upper limit of normal. The
albumin and clotting profiles were
normal. There was a positive antinuclear
antibody on serological testing, but no
evidence for viral hepatitis. Ultrasonography was non-contributory and a liver
biopsy was performed. Two typical
sections stained with haematoxylin and
eosin are shown (103a, 103b).
What is the diagnosis?

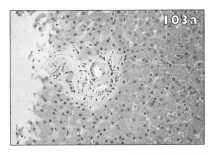

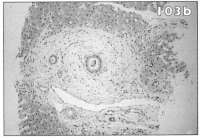

104 A barium enema from a 70-year-old man with acute bloody diarrhoea
and left hypochondrial pain is shown (104a). 104b shows a repeat study at 6
months after spontaneous recovery.
i. Describe the key of the first study.
What is the most likely diagnosis?
ii. What is the frequency of rectal
involvement?
iii. Is avoidance of surgery typical?

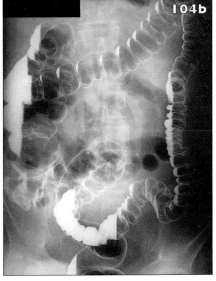

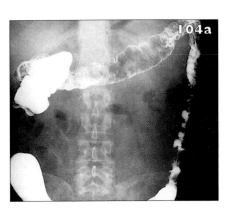

103 & 104: Answers

103 The characteristic lamellar fibrosis – onion skin effect – of primary sclerosing cholangitis is seen. Children present with a more hepatic illness than adults, and the coexistence of autoantibodies led to the incorrect belief previously that these children had a form of autoimmune chronic active hepatitis. Management is as for adults except that there often appears to be some response to steroid therapy.

104 i. Submucosal oedema and haemorrhage with segmental involvement of the splenic flexure and descending colon have produced 'thumb-printing', typical of ischaemic colitis (104a).
ii. Rectal involvement is unusual because of its good blood supply.
iii. Spontaneous resolution is typical.

Ischaemic colitis generally affects the watershed area of the two mesenteric arteries. The splenic flexure is therefore the most common site involved. Relatively elderly patients with evidence of ischaemic disease or low perfusion are at risk. An acute presentation with full recovery is common, although perforation and stricturing may occur. Surgery is reserved for those with peritonitis or fulminant colitis and for failure to settle.

105 A 52-year-old woman gives a 3-year history of abdominal discomfort and bloating. She has suffered from long-standing constipation. There has been some rectal bleeding but no weight loss. Her mother died of colonic carcinoma at age 56 years. Sigmoidoscopy was abnormal (105).
i. What does 105 show?
ii. Discuss the differential diagnosis.
iii. What other investigations are indicated?
iv. How should she be treated?

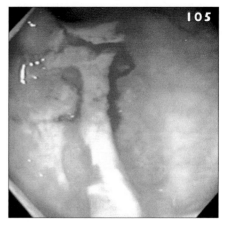

106 A 56-year-old salesman presents with a 1-year history of chronic diarrhoea, lethargy and weight loss. He has been taking non-prescription ibuprofen for joint pains. He does not drink or smoke and has a negative travel history. His wife reports that his memory is failing and that his work record has become unsatisfactory. Examination reveals him to be mildly febrile with a diffuse lymphadenopathy. A patchy skin pigmentation does not involve the buccal mucosa. There is a regurgitant murmur at the apex and a fullness is detected in the epigastrium. No hepatosplenomegaly is found. A Sudan stain performed on the stools is mildly positive. The haemoglobin is 10.7 g/dl, WBC count 12×10^9/l (12 000/mm^3) with a relative lymphopenia, and platelets 522×10^9/l (522 000/mm^3). The serum albumin is 2.4 g/dl. The ESR is 110 mm/h.
i. Discuss the differential diagnosis.
ii. A barium study demonstrates coarse folds in the proximal small bowel. A small-bowel biopsy is performed (106a, 106b). Comment on the histological findings.
iii. What is the diagnosis? Name the aetiological agent.
iv. Which disorders may mimic these histological features? Describe non-histological methods to assist in the diagnosis.
v. Comment on his memory lapses.
vi. Discuss treatment.

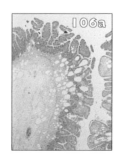
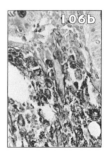

105 & 106: Answers

105 i. There is a large superficial linear ulcer in the rectum (**105**) with the appearances of the solitary rectal ulcer syndrome (SRUS).
ii. The differential diagnosis includes neoplasia, Crohn's disease, and viral infection (e.g. cytomegalovirus).
iii. SRUS is associated with disordered defaecation. A failure of relaxation of the pelvic floor muscles during normal straining results in an abnormally acute anorectal angle which hinders evacuation of the rectal contents. This predisposes to anterior mucosal prolapse, and ulceration. Histologically, fibrous tissue increases, and muscle fibres extend from the muscularis mucosae into the mucosa and between the crypts.
iv. Treatment includes the relief of constipation with bulking agents and/or stool softeners. Biofeedback may be helpful.

106 i. This man has a febrile, multisystem disorder probably involving the gut. Possibilities include lymphoma, sarcoidosis, HIV infection, collagen disorder, endocarditis and granulomatous disease. Chronic infection is less likely.
ii. The villi are clubbed and the lamina propria packed with macrophages staining positively with PAS. These inclusions tend to be rounded or sickle-shaped. The lacteals may also be dilated in this disorder (**106c**).
iii. Whipple's disease (caused by infection with *Tropheryma whippelii*).
iv. PAS-positive macrophages may also be seen in systemic histoplasmosis, macroglobulinaemia and *Mycobacterium avium* complex infection. In the last, bacilli are easily identified within the macrophages with acid-fast stains. Electron microscopy is useful in subtle Whipple's disease and may demonstrate numerous extracellular bacilli as well as phagocytosed bacilli in various stages of digestion within macrophages. Diagnosis may be confirmed by PCR.
v. Dementia, ophthalmoplegia and myoclonus are the most common manifestations of CNS involvement, which is almost universal at autopsy. CT and MRI may detect lesions but cerebrospinal fluid analysis rarely shows PAS-positive macrophages. Late CNS 'relapses' may be due to gliosis resulting from the original injury.
vi. Treatment should continue for at least 1 year and include an agent that crosses the blood–brain barrier in the presence of uninflamed meninges. Oral double-strength

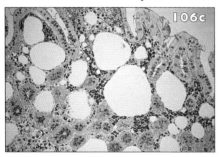

trimethoprim–sulphamethoxazole twice daily fulfils these criteria. Some precede this with a 2-week course of intramuscular penicillin and streptomycin. Chloramphenicol is used if there has been a failure to respond in the presence of CNS disease. Macrophages may persist for years after successful treatment.

107 This lesion (107) at the cardia was found in a 64-year-old patient being investigated for iron-deficiency anaemia.
i. What is it, and what is the aetiology?
ii. Where else may such a lesion be found?
iii. What treatment would you advocate?

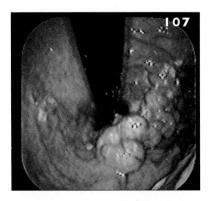

108 A 56-year-old alcoholic man was admitted with progressive epigastric pain, nausea and vomiting. His caloric intake for the previous 3 months had been

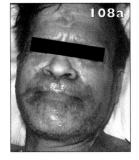

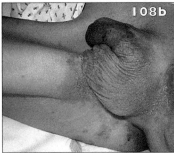

almost exclusively beer. He had previously had a partial gastrectomy with a Billroth II anastomosis. Upper gastrointestinal endoscopy on admission revealed stenosis at the previous surgery site. Parenteral nutrition was begun in an attempt to improve his nutritional status before surgery. However, a few days later he developed diarrhoea and skin lesions (108a, 108b).
i. Discuss the differential diagnosis of these skin lesions.
ii. Further blood work and a skin biopsy of an uninvolved area (108c) were performed. What is the patient's diagnosis and how may it be confirmed?
iii. What situations may predispose to this problem?
iv. What is the function of the deficient 'substance'?
v. Name other ways in which this clinical condition could present besides skin lesions.

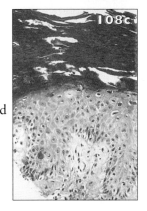

107 i. This is a varix, with a typical 'bunch of grapes' appearance. Gastric varices account for up to 10% of variceal bleeding episodes. Occasionally they may ooze slowly, resulting in anaemia. Collaterals between the portal and systemic venous circulations develop when the portal pressure exceeds 14 mmHg. Isolated gastric varices usually indicate splenic vein thrombosis resulting in segmental portal hypertension, but are more commonly found in association with oesophageal varices. Occasionally, gastric varices develop following obliteration of oesophageal varices.
ii. Varices are found in the oesophagus, subcardially, in the fundus and along the lesser curve in the stomach. They also develop around the spleen, in the rectum, and/or around the umbilicus as a caput medusa. Other sites include the left renal vein, the lumbar veins, and the ovarian or testicular veins.
iii. There is currently no consensus regarding treatment of gastric varices, but if not actively bleeding, they are probably best left alone. Initial haemostasis and rebleeding rates are poor after sclerotherapy. Newer treatments with adhesives or thrombin hold some promise. Banding may increase the rebleeding rate. The best course of management at present is probably to control the haemorrhage initially with balloon tamponade and vasoconstrictor agents, pending TIPSS (transjugular intrahepatic portosystemic stent shunting), surgical devascularization or shunting.
    In this patient, if the anaemia cannot be controlled with oral iron, elective TIPSS or surgical intervention may be indicated.

108 i. The differential diagnosis includes *Herpes simplex*, *Candida*, bacterial infections, and zinc, fatty acid and biotin deficiencies.
ii. The patient has zinc deficiency or acrodermatitis enteropathica. The acral distribution of skin lesions, which are erythematous, scaling, vesicopustular or eroded plaques, is typical. The skin biopsy demonstrates both hyperkeratosis and parakeratosis. Serum zinc level was 1.0 µg/ml (normal: 7–12 µg/ml). Skin lesions rapidly resolve with zinc supplementation. In situations of stress, trauma, infection or inflammation, a decrease in the serum zinc concentration occurs with sequestration in the liver. Thus, there is an internal redistribution rather than a true deficiency. A serum zinc concentration of 1.0 µg/ml is markedly low and reflects true deficiency.
iii. Poor dietary intake may predispose to zinc deficiency. Red meat is an excellent source of zinc, and beer contains virtually none. Increased urinary losses are seen following trauma or diabetes, increased faecal losses with diarrhoeal states, and increased cutaneous losses with burn injuries.
vi. Zinc is a cofactor for a number of enzymes that participate in metabolism. The intestine is only 20% efficient in absorbing zinc, so most ingested zinc is excreted in the stool.
v. Skin lesions or acrodermatitis occur in severe deficiency. Other manifestations include growth retardation, anorexia, poor wound healing, depressed night vision, hypogonadism, impaired immunity, diarrhoea, depressed mental function, and teratogenesis.

109 During a hot summer, a 59-year-old woman presented with vomiting and general malaise. Six months previously she had undergone resection of much of her small bowel after a spontaneous mesenteric vein thrombosis, leaving her with 60 cm of jejunum terminating in a stoma. She had been on anticoagulants and home parenteral nutrition. Because of the hot weather she had been drinking more than usual. Examination revealed an unwell woman, slightly confused. She was apyrexial but there was a tachycardia of 106 beats/min and hypotension (BP 100/70 mmHg lying, falling to 75/50 mmHg on sitting up). There were no signs of infection and the stoma appeared healthy and functional. Investigations revealed a low plasma sodium (116 mmol/l), high potassium (6.9 mmol/l) and substantial elevation of BUN (42 mmol/l; 59 mg/dl) and creatinine (330 μmol/l; 3.7 mg/dl). The INR was in the mid-therapeutic range at 3.2.
i. What has happened?
ii. What treatment is required?
iii. How can recurrence be avoided?

110 A 35-year-old man develops dyspnoea and a right pleural effusion after a severe attack of alcoholic pancreatitis. A litre of fluid is removed and is found to contain >20 000 iu/ml of amylase. The pleural fluid rapidly reaccumulates. Cytological examination of the fluid is negative for malignancy. A CT scan of the abdomen is performed (**110a**).
i. Describe the abnormalities in **110a**.
ii. What additional procedure may help to define the aetiology?
iii. What abnormality is revealed in **110b**?
iv. Suggest a management plan.
v. During his hospitalization, the patient develops ascites; the ascitic fluid is also rich in amylase. What might have occurred?

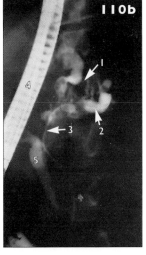

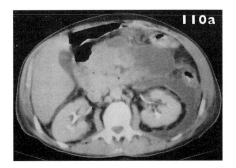

109 & 110: Answers

109 i. This patient has pre-renal azotaemia due to excessive losses from the jejunostomy. The hyponatraemia indicates a massive sodium deficit. The crisis was probably provoked by the hot weather, thirst reflecting a normal response to increased insensible losses. Unfortunately sodium (and therefore water) absorption in the jejunum can occur only against a small concentration gradient coupled to glucose absorption. When the luminal sodium content is below 90 mmol/l net secretion is usual. A stoma <100 cm from the duodenal–jejunal junction is insufficiently distal for a net absorptive state to be possible in most individuals. The stomal losses therefore bear a fairly steady sodium output of around 90 mmol/l. The additional fluids drunk because of thirst further dilute the luminal contents, exacerbating the secretory state, and fluid and sodium loss.
ii. Intravenous saline is required to reduce the potassium level rapidly. Specific intervention may be considered for worsening hyperkalaemia.
iii. In less compromised patients the use of oral rehydration solutions may be sufficient during hot weather, or for thirst of any cause. Opioids such as loperamide can also be useful. Intravenous saline during spells of unusually hot weather may be necessary.

110 i. The CT scan demonstrates a uniformly enlarged pancreas without a mass lesion or pseudocyst, consistent with oedematous pancreatitis.
ii. Pancreatography (ERCP) helps in view of the high amylase content of the pleural fluid.
iii. The pancreatogram reveals a pancreaticopleural fistula, an unusual complication of acute pancreatitis. This is the result of pancreatic duct rupture with consequent leakage of secretions outside the gland. Activation of proteolytic pancreatic enzymes results in local autodigestion of tissues. In general, these fistulae track into the chest through the crura of the diaphragm (1 = pancreatic–pleural fistula; 2 = pancreatic

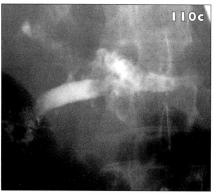

duct; 3 = ERCP catheter and guide wires; 4 = endoscope; 5 = bile duct).
iv. Although surgery is the definitive management, endoscopic stenting of the pancreatic duct across the leak occasionally allows the fistula to close. The use of octreotide may reduce pancreatic exocrine secretion. Ultimately, most patients with pancreaticopleural fistulae require surgery.
v. The development of pancreatic ascites suggests a pancreaticoperitoneal fistula. Pancreatography may demonstrate extravasation of contrast into the peritoneal cavity (110c).

111 A 50-year-old man presented with epigastric and right upper quadrant pain and a haematemesis. He had been on no medication, but was a smoker. There was tenderness in the upper abdomen but no other signs. He was not shocked and routine investigations were normal apart from a slightly elevated platelet count. Endoscopy was arranged (111).

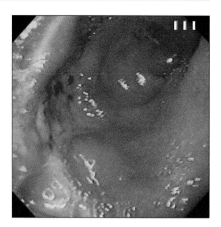

i. What is shown?
ii. What (other) signs indicate an increased risk of rebleeding?
iii. What major aetiological factor is implicated in this case?

112 A 24-year-old woman undergoing treatment for non-Hodgkin lymphoma develops lower abdominal discomfort associated with the passage of loose stools following her first cycle of chemotherapy. Stool examination is negative for faecal leukocytes, ova, parasites and *C. difficile* toxin, and routine bacterial culture is negative. The pain intensifies, becomes continuous, and the patient reports the onset of nausea and abdominal fullness. The stools continue to be non-bloody and liquid. Blood cultures are negative. Examination reveals that her temperature is 38.4°C, pulse 92/min regular. Respiratory and cardiovascular systems are normal and the abdomen is distended, tympanic without free fluid, and extremely tender to deep palpation in the right quadrants. There is a suggestion of peritonism over the tender area. Bowel sounds are diminished but high-pitched. Rectal examination is normal. The haemoglobin is 9.8 g/dl; WBC count 0.1×10^9/l (100/mm^3); and platelets 45×10^9/l (45 000/mm^3). The serum albumin is 21 g/l. A CT scan of the abdomen was performed (112).

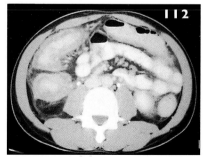

i. Comment on the radiological findings.
ii. Discuss the likely diagnoses.
iii. What is the most likely diagnosis and how may it be confirmed?
iv. What is the natural history of this disorder?
v. Comment on management of this patient.

111 & 112: Answers

111 i. There is a duodenal ulcer, with red spots indicative of recent bleeding and of a higher risk of rebleeding (**111**).
ii. Other 'stigmata' of recent bleeding include adherent clot over the ulcer, active continuing bleeding, and the presence of a visible vessel, each associated with a substantially increased risk of rebleeding. In this case, if the patient is not shocked and these signs are absent, the risk of rebleeding is low and it is often legitimate to discharge the patient from hospital immediately after the endoscopy.
iii. Although he is a smoker, the most likely aetiological factor (in the absence of a history of drugs damaging to the upper GI tract) is infection with *H. pylori*.

112 i. The CT scan demonstrates a markedly thickened caecum. There is no abscess, lymphadenopathy or ascites.
ii. The patient presents with diarrhoea and CT evidence for typhlitis. She has lymphoma and is immunosuppressed. An opportunistic infection due to *C. difficile* and cytomegalovirus must be excluded. Lymphomatous involvement of the bowel is possible but unlikely to present during treatment. Crohn's disease is also very unlikely to present during a state of T-cell suppression. There is no mass to suggest a submucosal haematoma, or skin rash to support a diagnosis of chemotherapy-induced graft-versus-host disease. Medications may occasionally be responsible for a drug-induced colitis. Ischaemia and diverticulitis are unusual at this age. The development of colitis, particularly involving the caecum (typhlitis), during a period of profound leukopenia is very suggestive of neutropenic colitis.
iii. Neutropenic colitis is a diagnosis of exclusion made in the setting of colitis and profound neutropenia, when other causes, particularly opportunistic infections, have been excluded. Patients are usually too ill to undergo colonoscopy. Pathological findings include ulceration, haemorrhage and secondary bacterial and fungal invasion. A gentle sigmoidoscopy may exclude overt inflammatory disease or pseudomembrane formation involving the distal colon, but usually has little to contribute.
iv. The colitis generally resolves rapidly once the neutropenia has been reversed; however, this is not invariable. Peritonism, progressive ileus, superinfection and perforation may occur and ultimately prove fatal.
v. Rapid reversal of the leukopenia by administration of recombinant granulocyte colony-stimulating factor is central to successful medical management. She should be kept nil per mouth, receive parenteral nutritional and broad-spectrum antimicrobial support. Frequently, clinical and radiographical monitoring are essential – until clinical resolution occurs. The presence of peritonism, progressive ileus and unremitting fever suggests impending perforation, and serious consideration to hemicolectomy must be given to pre-empt perforation, which is poorly tolerated. Some clinicians have advocated prophylactic colectomy before the administration of subsequent cycles of chemotherapy, as repeat episodes may occur with the accompanying neutropenia. However, early administration of colony-stimulating factor generally pre-empts such relapses.

113 An 11-month-old girl presents with a 1-month history of watery diarrhoea with no mucus or blood, occurring 3–6 times daily. There had been mild but persistent pyrexia and occasional vomiting. She had failed to gain weight., was fretful and slightly dehydrated with some loss of gluteal bulk. Otherwise, the examination was normal.
i. What is the likely diagnosis and its mechanism?
ii. What investigation is required to support this?

114 A 57-year-old engineer presents with a life-long history of painless constipation now unresponsive to laxatives. He was recently hospitalized with faecal impaction. He had a healthy diet, exercised daily and denied rectal bleeding or weight loss. Clinical examination showed mild abdominal distention. He could not expel a 50 ml water-filled balloon from the rectum. A barium enema is performed (114a).
i. Comment on this investigation (114a).
ii. What is the diagnosis?
iii. How would you confirm this diagnosis?
iv. Comment on the histopathology in 114b and 114c.
v. What is the pathogenesis of this condition?
vi. Discuss treatment options.

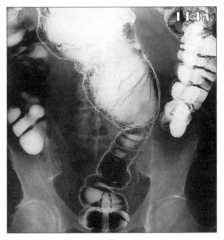

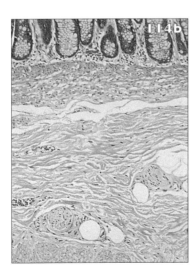

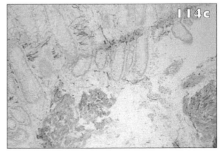

113 i. This proved to be post-enteritis syndrome following an episode of gastroenteritis; the gastroenteritis generally goes on to intermittent or chronic diarrhoea for more than 2 weeks with or without failure to gain weight on the return to a normal diet. The WHO defines chronic diarrhoea as three or more liquid stools per 24 hours, lasting for 14 days or longer. It may be due to persistence of the original infecting organism, reinfection with another pathogen, or sensitization to food antigens causing persistence of small intestinal mucosal damage.
ii. Further microbiological investigation of the stools, including viral studies, is required. Persistent infections most often associated with the post-enteritis syndrome are enteropathogenic *E. coli*, *Giardia* and *Campylobacter* species. Small-bowel biopsy may be required. The prognosis is generally good.

114 i. This demonstrates massive dilatation of the sigmoid colon. The rectum is normal but in the mid-sigmoid region, the luminal diameter changes suddenly from a normal-size rectum to a dilated sigmoid colon, without obvious luminal obstruction.
ii. Hirschsprung's disease.
iii. Confirmatory tests include a full-thickness rectal biopsy with staining for neural ganglia and acetylcholinesterase stain for neural hyperplasia. Anorectal manometry is also useful. Normally, rectal distention induces reflex relaxation of the internal anal sphincter – the rectoanal inhibitory reflex. This reflex depends on the integrity of the myenteric plexus. In Hirschsprung's disease, this reflex is absent.
iv. 114b shows haematoxylin and eosin staining of a rectal biopsy demonstrating absence of ganglion cells in the submucosa. 114c shows special staining for acetylcholinesterase, and shows abnormal, thick branches of neural fibres in the lamina propria. These features are pathognomonic of Hirschsprung's disease.
v. Hirschsprung's disease is a developmental disorder characterized by the absence of ganglion cells in the myenteric and submucosal plexus of the distal colon. Typically, a short segment of rectum or rectosigmoid is involved. Aganglionosis occurs because of the arrest of caudad migration of cells from the neural crest that were destined to develop as the myenteric nerve plexus. Hence, the aganglionic segment is always distal and is in continuity with the anus, and its length variable. This congenital defect occurs in approximately 1 in 5000 live births, is more common in males, and is usually recognized during infancy. The aganglionic segment fails to relax and permit passage of stool. Hence, the normal segment of bowel proximal to the zone of aganglionosis becomes dilated. Recent studies have shown that the primary neurophysiological abnormality is the absence of nitric oxide-producing cells, important for internal anal sphincter relaxation.
vi. Surgery offers definitive cure. The chief goal is to remove the aganglionic segment.

115 This lesion (**115a**) appeared on the outer aspect of the shin of a 68-year-old woman. She had generally enjoyed good health apart from episodic bouts of bloody diarrhoea which would settle spontaneously.
i. What is the lesion?
ii. Name three conditions with which it is associated.
iii. What is the likely underlying diagnosis in this patient?
iv. What other skin condition is also commonly seen with this diagnosis?

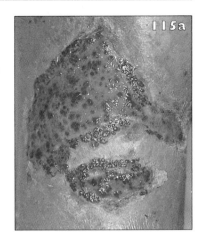

116 A 47-year-old woman underwent a jejunoileal bypass procedure 8 years previously for morbid obesity. She now has a 2-day history of mental status change, unsteadiness and slurring of speech. She does not drink or smoke, takes loperamide for diarrhoea, and has used aspirin for the past 4 weeks. She is found to be afebrile without dehydration and normal haemodynamics. The respiratory, cardiovascular and abdominal examinations are normal apart from the scars of her prior surgery. She is obtunded without neck stiffness or localizing signs. Fundoscopy is normal. The blood count, glucose, urea nitrogen, creatinine, chest radiograph and head CT scan are within normal limits. There are no ketones in the urine and the plasma salicylate level is low. The laboratory results are provided in the table.
i. Comment on the laboratory data.
ii. What diagnosis needs to be considered, and how may this be confirmed?
iii. Discuss the pathogenesis of this disorder.
iv. Discuss treatment.

Investigation	Result
Sodium	137 mmol/l
Potassium	3.3 mmol/l
Chloride	100 mmol/l
Bicarbonate	12 mmol/l
Arterial blood pH	7.29
Arterial blood gases	
pCO_2	22 mmHg
pO_2	102 mmHg

115 & 116: Answers

115 i. Pyoderma gangrenosum.
ii. Inflammatory bowel disease (IBD),
paraproteinaemias, vasculitides, haematological
malignancies, idiopathic in 30% of cases.
iii. Ulcerative colitis.
iv. Skin manifestations occur in up to 20% of
patients, especially pyoderma gangrenosum and
erythema nodosum, occurring in around 5%.
Dermatitis, erythema, psoriasis, carcinoma,
urticaria, pityriasis, lupus, vitiligo, ecchymosis,
and other drug-related lesions also occur.

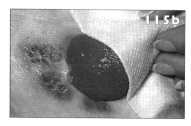
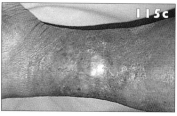

Pyoderma begins as a discrete pustule or
erythematous papule progressing to a deeper
undermined ulcer with a characteristic
violaceous edge. It most commonly affects the
pre-tibial region, but can occur at almost any
site, particularly sites of previous trauma (**115b**).

The histology is characterized by endothelial injury with fibrinoid necrosis of the
blood vessels and marked infiltration inflammatory infiltrate.

Pyoderma may precede the onset of IBD, run an independent course, respond
poorly to resection of diseased intestine, or develop after panproctocolectomy for
ulcerative colitis.

Erythema nodosum presents as tender, red nodules on the anterior surface of the
lower extremities, often associated with arthritis. The lesions generally occur during
bouts of colonic disease activity and usually respond to therapy directed at the colon;
115c shows scarring left after treatment of **115a** with steroids and
immunosuppressants. Cyclosporine and/or dapsone may also be useful.

116 i. The patient has an anion-gap metabolic acidosis, indicating the presence of
unmeasured anions. Hypokalaemia is probably secondary to the diarrhoea. Uraemia,
ketoacidosis, hyperglycaemia, and other ingested toxins have been excluded.
ii. This syndrome is a complication of surgical procedures that facilitate the
overgrowth of D-lactate-producing Gram-positive organisms. The elevated plasma D-
lactate level is diagnostic. The L-isomer may be normal.
iii. While L-lactate is a product of anaerobic metabolism, D-lactate is the result of
bacterial metabolism of carbohydrate by isomer-specific D-lactate dehydrogenase
activity. A neuropsychiatric syndrome may become manifest, sometimes years after
the surgery, once a critical threshold is attained. Symptoms include headache,
alterations in affect, delirium, visual disturbances, dysarthria, ataxia and cranial
nerve palsies.
iv. Treatment includes carbohydrate restriction and non-absorbable antibiotics.
Transient improvement may be the result of reduced intake.

117 A 3-year-old boy has been passing a 'bulky stool like cooking oil' since birth. He was born at term after a normal pregnancy with a birth weight on the 90th centile. Meconium was passed within 24 hours. He was breast-fed until 4 months and then on a cows' milk formula. Solids were introduced at 6 months. His family doctor had twice treated a cough with antibiotics. There was no family history of relevance. Examination revealed pectus excavatum and protuberant abdomen. His growth chart is shown in 117.
i. What is the most likely diagnosis?
ii. What are the most useful investigations here?

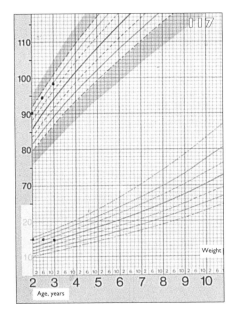

118 A 46-year-old man with chronic renal failure on haemodialysis, presents with a 6-month history of a 9 kg (20 lb) pound weight loss, nausea, intermittent vomiting, and an inability to tolerate solid food. He reports epigastric discomfort and early satiety. He has experienced occasional loose stools, particularly in the evenings, and episodes of faecal incontinence. He denies any history of peptic ulcer disease. He has a 20-year history of type I diabetes. On examination, he is thinly built with mild pedal oedema and a blood pressure of 160/100 mmHg. Haemoglobin is 9.2 g/dl; haematocrit 30%; mean corpuscular volume 92 fl; BUN 28.4 mmol/l (40 mg/dl); creatinine 212 µmol/l (2.4 mg/dl); electrolytes normal; glucose 13.1 mmol/l (236 mg/dl); albumin 35 g/l. A barium examination is performed (118a).

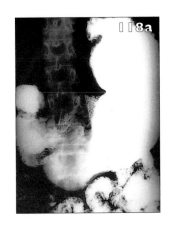

i. What does the 118a demonstrate?
ii. What are the diagnostic possibilities?
iii. Describe additional relevant investigations.
iv. What is the significance of the diarrhoea?
v. Discuss management.

117 i. The most likely diagnosis is cystic fibrosis.
ii. Investigations should include sweat test, chest radiograph, pancreatic assessment, and analysis for the CFTR cystic fibrosis gene mutation.

Pancreatic insufficiency, which affects about 85% of children with cystic fibrosis, may be obvious from the positive faecal fat stain, which occurs when the lipase secretion falls below 10%. About 12% of cases present neonatally with meconium ileus and small-bowel obstruction, which results from the collection of viscid intraluminal contents, usually in the terminal ileum. Meglumine diatrizoate enema may be both diagnostic and therapeutic, but surgery is occasionally required. Fibrosing colonopathy may occur in children treated with high-dose pancreatic enzyme supplements, characterized by submucosal fibrosis causing stenosis, and may be responsible for constipation. Rectal prolapse affects up to 20% of cases. The fat malabsorption makes attention to the fat-soluble vitamins particularly important. Clinically, overt liver disease develops in 4% of cases and is the cause of death in 2% (from liver failure or portal hypertensive bleeding). Microscopic evidence of small bile duct obstruction occurs in 50% of cases.

118 i. 118a demonstrates a markedly enlarged stomach, but no evidence of intestinal obstruction.
ii. The features are consistent with gastroparesis. Stenosis as a result of peptic ulceration of the pyloric area or duodenum could result in emptying difficulties. Other processes including malignancies and extrinsic compression may produce similar features.
iii. Endoscopy excludes an obstructed gastric outlet. A stomach full of debris (**118b**) may make examination difficult. Gastric emptying may be quantitatively evaluated by a scintigraphy. Antroduodenojejunal manometry may identify dysmotility.
iv. The presence of diarrhoea in a diabetic is suggestive of an autonomic neuropathy, particularly if other causes have been excluded. This disorder is precipitated by

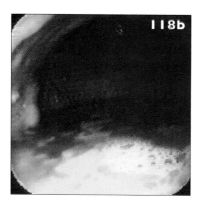

bacterial overgrowth and may be confirmed by jejunal culture, hydrogen breath testing, or empiric antibiotic trial. A faecal fat stain should be performed to screen for steatorrhoea.
v. Prokinetic drugs may improve gastric emptying, but may aggravate the diarrhoea. The nutritional needs of patients must be met and occasionally surgery may be necessary. Insertion of a jejunal feeding tube may be considered for intractable cases and is preferable to home parenteral nutrition. Antimicrobials may be useful in treating bacterial overgrowth.

119 i. What does this investigation show (119a)?
ii. What is the significance of the negative CLO (rapid urease) test (119b)?
iii. What further investigations are considered in this patient who had previously been asymptomatic and had taken no medication at the time of investigation?

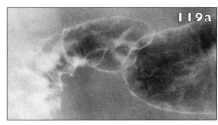

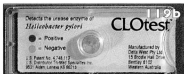

120 A 20-year-old student develops cramping abdominal pain, diarrhoea and vomiting soon after returning from vacation. He is admitted for rehydration in view of postural hypotension, a blood urea nitrogen of 24 mmol/l (34 mg/dl) [normal, 7.1–14.2 mmol/l (10–20 mg/dl)] and a creatinine of 124 µmol/l (1.4 mg/dl) [normal, 71–115 µmol/l (0.8–1.3 mg/dl)]. He and friends ate at fast-food outlets during their vacation and one also developed diarrhoea after coming home. His dehydration responds to intravenous fluids but the diarrhoea persists and becomes grossly bloody within 24 hours. Stool specimens for routine culture, ova and parasites are normal, although white cells are identified on Wright's stain. Flexible sigmoidoscopy reveals haemorrhagic colitis throughout (120a) with biopsies revealing severe acute colitis without crypt

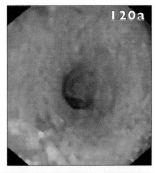

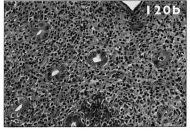

architecture distortion (120b). His hospital course is further complicated by worsening renal function (creatinine 230 µmol/l; 2.6 mg/dl) on day 3, anaemia (haemoglobin 8.1 g/dl) and thrombocytopenia [platelet count 65×10^9/l (65 000/mm^3)].
i. What is the likely diagnosis?
ii. Discuss other possible aetiologies.
iii. Does his friend with diarrhoea have the same illness?
iv. How may the diagnosis be confirmed?
v. Should he receive antibiotics, steroids, or both?

111

119 & 120: Answers

119 i. The barium meal (**119a**) shows an ulcer in the duodenal bulb.
ii. The negative urease test (**119b**) indicates that current infection with *Helicobacter pylori* is unlikely. About 95% of duodenal ulcers occurring in the absence of exposure to non-steroidal anti-inflammatories are caused (at least in part) by *H. pylori*, but not this one. The following should be considered: Zollinger–Ellison syndrome, Crohn's disease, pancreatic ectasia, hypercalcaemia, sarcoidosis, or hereditary excess of functional parietal cells.
iii. Further investigation might include *H. pylori* serology or urea breath testing (to confirm that the patient really is *H. pylori*-free), biopsies of the ulcer, fasting gastrin, serum calcium, Kveim test, and gastric acid output tests.

120 i. This presentation is highly suggestive of enterohaemorrhagic *E. coli* (EHEC) infection due to serotype O157:H7, a virulent pathogen that elaborates Shiga-like cytotoxins that damage epithelial and endothelial cells. Infection is generally acquired from eating improperly cooked ground beef. After a short incubation period, patients experience severe cramping, with diarrhoea and vomiting in 50% of cases. A low-grade fever may be present. Bloody diarrhoea usually begins 1–3 days later. The clinical course is self-limiting but complications may occur, such as haemolytic uraemic syndrome and thrombotic thrombocytopenic purpura.
ii. Shigellosis, *Campylobacter* infection and salmonellosis may present similarly, but are easily cultured with standard techniques. Amoebiasis may be identified by direct examination of stools and serologies. *De novo* inflammatory bowel disease may occasionally present acutely. Ischaemic colitis would be unusual in a patient with no risk factors. *C. difficile* colitis usually occurs in relation to antibiotic exposure and, the stools are typically non-bloody.
iii. More than one case is typically identified if the infection is acquired from a restaurant or social function.
iv. Conventional stool cultures are invariably negative for pathogens. *E. coli* O157:H7 is cultured using sorbitol–MacConkey agar.
v. Treatment is generally supportive. Antibiotics are of no proved benefit. Patients with complications need to be carefully monitored since fatalities may occur in these subgroups and haemodialysis or exchange transfusion may be required. The most important method of preventing infection is to ensure that ground beef is well cooked.

121 A barium study (121) was performed in a
50-year-old male with abdominal pain, vomiting
and fever.
i. What abnormalities are seen and what is the
most likely diagnosis?
ii. What further investigations are required?

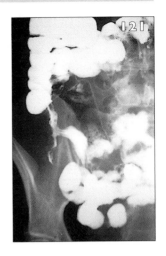

122 A 29-year-old man with a 5-year history of HIV positivity and a history
of pneumocystis pneumonia 1 year previously, now presents with weight loss,
mild periumbilical pain, and diarrhoea. There is minimal association of
symptoms with eating meals. A physical examination reveals diffuse muscle
wasting, but is otherwise non-focal. Routine stool studies are negative for
faecal leukocytes, *Clostridium difficile* toxin, ova and parasites, and bacterial
culture. An upper endoscopy with
small-bowel biopsy is performed and
demonstrates 'dots' adherent to the
brush-border lining (122a). Stools
stained with a modified acid-fast stain
demonstrate the features seen in 122b.
Flexible sigmoidoscopy with rectal
biopsy is unremarkable.
i. Which pathogen is present?
ii. Which complications may occur?
iii. Comment on antimicrobial
therapies available for treatment of
the identified pathogen.
iv. Which additional therapies are
available to attempt to control
diarrhoeal symptoms?
v. Which other pathogens may be
responsible for diarrhoea in patients
with AIDS?

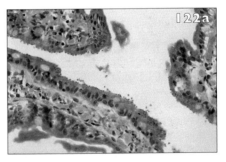

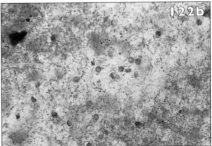

121 & 122: Answers

121 i. 121 shows stricturing and irregularity of the ileum with a deformed ileocaecal junction and a contracted and deformed caecum with ulcerated mucosa. Intestinal tuberculosis is the most likely diagnosis on radiological grounds. Crohn's disease, intestinal lymphoma, peritoneal carcinomatosis and actinomycosis are possible differentials.
ii. Routine investigation for tuberculosis (Mantoux test, chest radiograph, gastric washings) may confirm the diagnosis as may histological or microbiological study of biopsies obtained at colonoscopy, especially if terminal ileal samples can be obtained. It is likely that polymerase chain reaction-based technology will provide a new means to DNA-based diagnosis.

Intestinal tuberculosis most commonly affects the caecum (in >85% of cases) but no site is exempt. It occurs increasingly more commonly, especially in patients with HIV infection, which this patient proved to have. The disease is usually predominantly ulcerative (in 60% of cases) but hypertrophic and ulcerohypertrophic forms occur. It can be very difficult to distinguish from Crohn's disease as half of all patients with abdominal tuberculosis have a normal chest radiograph. Positive tissue cultures, or the presence of caseation in granulomas are relatively rarely found but are conclusive. Therapeutic trials with antituberculous therapy may prove helpful.

122 i. Cryptosporidia are seen adherent to the intestinal brush-border surface. The parasite is also seen in the specially stained stool specimen.
ii. *Cryptosporidium* species are responsible for 10–20% of cases of AIDS-associated diarrhoea in the US and up to 55% of cases in developing nations. Cryptosporidiosis carries a significant mortality rate when the CD4+ count falls below 50. It has been associated with a papillitis of the ampulla of Vater (resulting in pancreatitis and bile duct obstruction), acalculous cholecystitis, and infection of the biliary ductal epithelium resulting in sclerosing cholangitis.
iii. *Cryptosporidium* is particularly resistant to antibiotic therapy. Macrolide antibiotics (e.g. spiramycin, azithromycin) and paromomycin have been utilized with variable results.
iv. The addition of bulking agents (e.g. psyllium) may decrease the frequency of bowel movements. A variety of antimotility agents may provide symptomatic relief, including loperamide, diphenoxylate, paregoric, codeine and tincture of opium. Octreotide has been demonstrated to reduce stool frequency and volume dramatically when administered subcutaneously in doses of 250 µg or 500 µg every 8 hours. A trial should be considered in patients who do not respond to antimotility agents. Occasionally, intravenous fluid and nutritional supplementation become necessary.
v. Other small bowel pathogens include: *Isospora belli*, microsporidia, *Giardia lamblia*, *Strongyloides*, *Mycobacterium avium*, *M. tuberculosis* and invasive bacterial pathogens. HIV itself appears to infect enterocytes and cause a diarrhoeal illness. Cytomegalovirus and *Entamoeba histolytica* infection may be responsible for colitis. Herpes simplex virus typically causes a proctitis marked by anorectal pain, tenesmus and occasional diarrhoea.

123 A 74-year-old woman underwent a flexible sigmoidoscopy for investigation of change in bowel habit. She had a long history of constipation, but for the preceding 6 months had complained of persistent diarrhoea. 123 shows the endoscopic appearance.
i. What is the diagnosis?
ii. What medications is she likely to be taking?
iii. What is the prognosis?

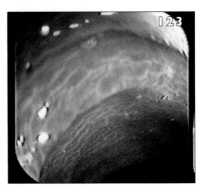

124 A 35-year-old schoolteacher complains of epigastric discomfort towards the end of the day and wakes him at night, generally between 2 and 4 a.m. It is relieved by eating biscuits and taking an over-the-counter antacid preparation. He is under considerable stress at work. There has been no loss of appetite, loss of weight, vomiting or change in bowel movements. He recalls a similar discomfort a few months previously that lasted a few weeks. He has not taken any other medications. He smokes fewer than five cigarettes per day and does not take any alcohol. Physical examination is normal apart from non-specific epigastric tenderness. The stools test negative for the presence of occult blood. Haematological data are given in the table.
i. What are the diagnostic possibilities?
ii. What further work-up is appropriate at this stage?
iii. How should he be treated?
iv. How should he be monitored?

Investigation	Result
Haemoglobin	13.5 g/dl
MCV	89.6 fl
WBC	7.9×10^9/l (7900/mm³)
ESR	2 mm/h
BUN	10.7 mmol/l (15 mg/dl)
Albumin	45 g/l (4.5 g/dl)
SGPT (ALT)	22 u/l
ALP	76 u/l
Amylase	54 iu/l

123 i. The diagnosis is melanosis coli. This classic endoscopic appearance (**123**) has been compared with tiger or crocodile skin. The colonic coloration varies from light brown to black and is due to lipofuscin deposition. The pigment may originate from degenerating cell constituents.

ii. Three-quarters of reported patients with melanosis coli use anthraquinone laxatives (e.g. senna, aloe, frangula). In most cases the pigmentation is totally reversible over a period of 9–12 months once the offending drug is stopped. The age of reported patients varies, but it is often a condition of older adults.

iii. Melanosis coli is generally considered to be a benign condition; however, it has been reported in association with colonic carcinoma via an unknown mechanism. Areas containing inflammation, neoplasia, regenerating epithelium or polyps do not contain pigment and hence any pink area seen at endoscopy is biopsied to exclude malignancy.

124 i. The history, nature of the discomfort, relationship to food, and position of the pain is highly suggestive of an acid peptic disorder – with peptic ulcer disease being the most likely. The periodicity (suggestive of spontaneous alleviation and relapse) also supports this diagnosis. Stress as a cause for functional dyspepsia is also possible. The absence of heartburn does not support a diagnosis of GORD despite the nocturnal symptoms. Gastritis is another possibility. Pancreatitis or biliary disease is unlikely.

ii. The absence of any alarm symptoms (e.g. bleeding, anaemia, weight loss, vomiting, dysphagia) in this young man, who is far more likely to have peptic ulcer disease than a malignancy, mitigates against any further investigations being performed at this time. However, algorithms for the work-up of dyspepsia are currently developed which incorporate a serum antibody test for *Helicobacter pylori* being performed early on in the management.

All other investigations must be considered with reserve, but may include an upper endoscopy, barium study and/or another abdominal imaging modality. The cost-effectiveness of empiric strategies for the treatment of dyspepsia remains controversial, with many clinicians citing the high relapse rate of symptoms following initial improvement (incidence >50% in many studies) as a reason to investigate early rather than later. Older patients have an increased incidence of serious disorders and should not receive empiric or symptomatic treatment indefinitely.

iii. Empiric therapy, employing an H2-receptor antagonist is appropriate treatment. A patient testing positive for *H. pylori* may receive a regimen including antimicrobial therapy for the eradication of this organism at this stage.

iv. Patients receiving empiric therapy for the treatment of dyspepsia are followed up after 2 weeks to evaluate response. Treatment is continued for at least 6 weeks in those who respond completely.

125 A 30-year-old woman underwent gastroscopy (125) for recurrent heartburn.
i. What is the main lesion?
ii. What complication has occurred?
iii. How should she be treated?

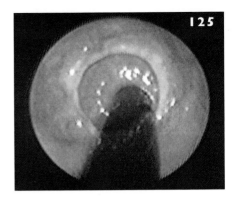

126 A 39-year-old woman gives a 4-year history of worsening faecal incontinence. She passes a formed stool twice a day. However, she has marked urgency with frank incontinence when she loses the entire motion about once a fortnight. She also reports passive leakage of faecal liquid and needs to wear a pad. She is socially disabled by her symptoms and has stopped working because of them. She has no urinary symptoms. Previously, she has had phenol injection of second-degree haemorrhoids 5 and 9 years previously. Four years ago she had a lateral sphincterotomy for anal fissure. She has had two vaginal deliveries, the first of which entailed forceps extraction. She is receiving no medication. General examination showed a reserved woman with no abnormality. There was an old episiotomy scar and poor anal sphincter tone. Haemorrhoids were present at proctoscopy. Anal sphincter manometry showed a resting pressure of $32\,cmH_2O$ (normal $89–109\,cmH_2O$) and voluntary contraction pressure of $40\,cmH_2O$ (normal $88–124\,cmH_2O$). 126 shows the appearances of her endoanal ultrasound scan (the anal canal is the circular structure in the middle of the image, anterior to the right).

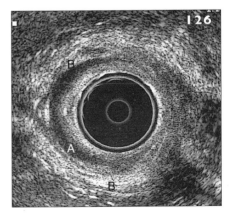

i. Identify structures A and B in 126.
ii. Comment on the abnormalities in the ultrasound.
iii. What is the likely aetiology of her faecal incontinence?
iv. What is the appropriate management of her incontinence?
v. How should any subsequent pregnancies be managed?

125 & 126: Answers

125 i. This is a small, sliding hiatus hernia (125) as seen with the endoscope in a 'J-position' which, as the name suggests, allows the endoscopist to look back long the shaft of the endoscope.
ii. The complication is the white ring, known as a Schatski ring, which is small here but may be large enough to cause dysphagia and require endoscopic (or radiological) dilatation.
iii. Many practitioners would treat her with an initial course of a proton pump inhibitor, followed by therapy tailored at the severity of her symptoms for recurrent symptoms, using antacids, H2-receptor antagonists, proton pump inhibitors or a prokinetic agent. Failure to respond to medical therapy is an indication for anti-reflux surgery.

126 i. 'A' is the internal sphincter; 'B' is the external sphincter.
ii. There is gross disruption of both the internal and external sphincters anteriorly.
iii. This is obstetric damage associated with the use of forceps. Her prior haemorrhoid surgery is probably unrelated to her faecal incontinence; following her lateral sphincterotomy any defect in the internal sphincter should be lateral whereas in this case it is anterior. Passive faecal incontinence is a symptom of internal anal sphincter damage (smooth muscle) and urge incontinence typically originates from external sphincter dysfunction (striated muscle). The most important factor in the development of sphincter damage appears to be use of forceps (four out of five cases); vacuum suction delivery causes damage in about one in five cases, and spontaneous delivery in one in six cases. Sphincter damage only causes defaecatory symptoms in about half of patients sustaining such obstetric injury. In the case of deliveries resulting in third-degree obstetric tears, the rate of incontinence is about 33% at 6 months post-partum.
iv. Endoanal ultrasound helps to localize the defect and thus delineate surgical repair, usually anterior overlap repair. No specific remedy is available for internal anal sphincter dysfunction but passive faecal incontinence tends to improve following surgical repair.

Loperamide is helpful in passive and urge faecal incontinence in the main part by providing the patient with confidence to lead as normal a life as possible with this disorder which can be socially disabling. Careful titration of the dose (easier using the suspension) should be stressed to avoid constipation, especially if the patient has irritable bowel-type symptoms.

Anal plugs made of polyurethane sponge with a water-soluble coat are of limited effectiveness. Behavioural biofeedback therapy has been reported as effective in patients with sphincter rupture. Simple continence advice should also be offered (use of pads and barrier creams, regular hygiene, etc.).
v. She should have a Caesarean section for any subsequent deliveries.

127 A 46-year-old woman presents with a 6-month history of intermittent rectal bleeding after bowel movements with blood on the stool and tissue, and in the toilet bowl. She has felt a soft, sometimes tender, swelling at the anal area which disappears when she stops bearing down, but recently she has had to apply pressure directly. She has been taking a mild laxative. Her appetite and weight are well preserved. There is no family history of colorectal neoplasia. Physical examination demonstrates a lesion (127a).

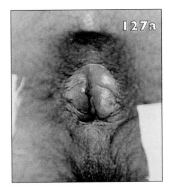

i. What is the diagnosis?
ii. What additional information may be required?
iii. Discuss complications of the underlying disorder.
iv. Describe applicable treatment modalities.

128 A 37-year-old woman with chronic alcohol abuse presents with a large haematemesis. Examination reveals no stigmata of chronic liver disease. She is pale and vasoconstricted with a blood pressure of 94/45 mmHg and a heart rate of 122/min. The abdomen is not distended, but there is tenderness to deep palpation in the right upper quadrant. The liver is not enlarged and there is no ascites. Blood count reveals a haemoglobin of 9.9 g/dl; white blood count 5.5×10^9/l (5500/mm³); and platelet count 89×10^9/l (89 000/mm³). Serum albumin, liver enzymes, PT and PTT are normal. Upper endoscopy reveals active haemorrhage from an elongated, tortuous fundic 'fold,' consistent with a varix (128a). The oesophagus and oesophagogastric junction are well seen and are normal.

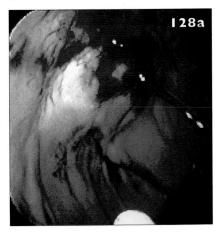

i. What is the endoscopic diagnosis?
ii. Discuss the likely pathogenesis.
iii. Comment on treatment of the bleeding.
iv. Discuss additional investigations that may be indicated.

127 i. Examination demonstrates the presence of external and third-degree internal haemorrhoids with sites of recent haemorrhage (boxes).
ii. Proctoscopic examination confirms their presence, but may be painful. Flexible sigmoidoscopy allows inspection of the haemorrhoids by retroflexion (**127b**). However, a complete colon evaluation is performed in patients at-risk for other

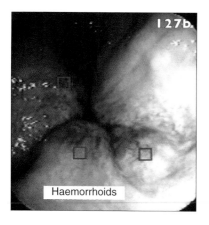

lesions. It is important to distinguish haemorrhoidal protrusion from true rectal prolapse.
iii. Bleeding is common, but anaemia unusual. Painful thrombosis, prolapse (which may be irreducible), pruritus and soiling may occur.
iv. Treatment consists of bulking agents and stool softeners. Anti-inflammatory suppositories or creams may be useful. Pain may respond to sitz baths. An ablative procedure may be necessary when symptoms persist. Options include photocoagulation, sclerosant injection, rubber-band ligation, or surgical excision.

128 i. The features are consistent with bleeding due to fundic varices.
ii. Isolated gastric varices (absence of associated oesophageal varices) may be due to chronic liver disease or splenic vein thrombosis. The splenic vein traverses the posterior margin of the pancreas, and is susceptible to both inflammatory and neoplastic processes.
iii. The circulation must be maintained. Vasopressin or octreotide may be used to decrease portal pressure. Sclerotherapy (**128b**), banding and combination therapy

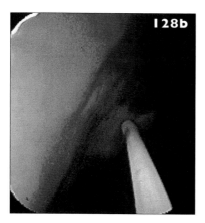

employing both modalities have variable success. Injection of adhesive agents is undergoing evaluation. Oesophagogastric balloon tamponade is seldom successful, and surgery is often necessary.
iv. Accurate diagnosis is essential as splenectomy is curative and portosystemic shunting unnecessary when splenic vein thrombosis is the cause. Absent splenic vein flow, retrograde venous drainage towards the splenic hilum, and the presence of thrombus may be detected by angiography with venous phase radiography, CT scanning with the use of intravenous contrast, magnetic resonance imaging, or Doppler sonography.

129 Match **i–vi** with the appropriate function **a–e** regarding gut immunity.

i. M (microfold) cell.   a. Synthesis and secretion of IgA.

ii. Peyer's patch.   b. Selection and transportation of antigen.

iii. Lamina propria.   c. T-cell with cytolytic function.

iv. J-chain.   d. Processing of ingested antigen.

v. Intraepithelial lymphocyte.   e. Transport and stabilization of polymeric IgA.

vi. Secretory component.

130 A 73-year-old woman has a 6-month history of weight loss, progressive abdominal distention, bloating and constipation alternating with diarrhoea, and moderately severe heartburn. She has noticed some 'tightness' of her hands. The facial and digital appearances are shown in **130a** and **130b**, respectively. On examination, she has a distended abdomen with sluggish bowel sounds, minimal abdominal tenderness and hyperresonance to percussion. The haemoglobin is 13.5 g/dl; lipase 39 iu/l; albumin 31 g/l; BUN 4.3 mmol/l (6 mg/dl); and creatinine 88 μmol/l (1.0 mg/dl). Liver enzymes and electrolytes are normal.

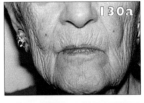
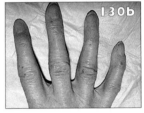

i. Comment on the facial and hand appearances.

ii. What is the diagnosis?

iii. Comment on aetiology, other organ involvement, and confirming this diagnosis.

iv. Comment on the manometric tracings in **130c**.

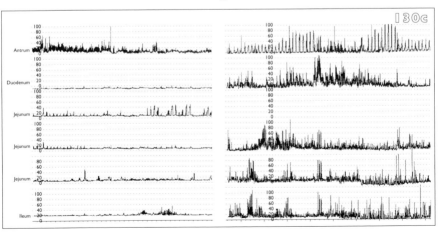

129 i. (b) The M cell is an elongated cell located in the dome epithelium. It selects and transports large macromolecules and microorganisms for processing in the underlying lymphoid follicular area – this leads to the development of a cellular recognition system.

ii. (d) The Peyer's patch is an organized lymphoid follicle, consisting of mainly precursor B-cells and a germinal centre. Lymphocytes and macrophages in the dome area, in conjunction with antigens (that have passed through the M cell from the lumen) prime lymphocytes. These activated lymphocytes (lymphoblasts) travel via lymphatics to secretory mucosal sites. IgA-bearing lymphoblasts predominate.

iii. (a) The lamina propria is the effector limb of the gut-associated lymphoid tissue (GALT) system. The synthesis and secretion of dimeric IgA by plasma cells in the lamina propria is the major protective mechanism of the gastrointestinal tract. This antibody is the most abundant antibody. IgA complexes to luminal antigen, neutralizing or bonding bacteria, viruses, etc.

iv. (e) The J chain is a polypeptide produced by the plasma cell that joins two IgA monomers to form a dimeric structure, and participates in transport of IgA across the intestinal epithelial cell.

v. (c) The intraepithelial lymphocytes are the first line of defence against epithelial events and appear to function biologically as cytolytic effectors (CD8+ cells). Their numbers are increased in coeliac disease, AIDS, protozoal infections, and graft-versus-host disease.

vi. None. Secretory component facilitates transmembrane transport of IgA, and also serves to protect it against luminal digestion.

130 i. Telangiectasia are seen on the cheeks, around the lips, on the forefingers and nail bed. The skin is shiny and demonstrates sclerodactyly.

ii. Systemic sclerosis.

iii. Systemic sclerosis is an autoimmune disorder. The diagnosis is supported by a biopsy of the skin, oesophagus or synovia. Antinuclear antibody is positive in most patients. Anticentromere antibody is sensitive and specific for the CREST syndrome (Calcinosis, Raynaud's phenomenon, Esophageal dysmotility, Sclerodactyly and Telangiectasia). SCL-70 antibody is specific and positive in 25% of cases. The ESR is normal in one-third of cases and elevated in the remainder. Small-intestinal involvement may cause dysmotility and bacterial overgrowth. Oesophageal involvement may cause severe reflux with stricturing. Renal involvement is responsible for recurrent urinary tract infections. Progressive pulmonary fibrosis and pneumonitis may occur.

iv. 130c shows postprandial antroduodenojejunal manometry, in a normal individual (left) and the patient (right). The normal 'fed response' consists of phasic contractions at three cycles per minute in the antrum and 11 cycles per minute in the duodenum and jejunum with an amplitude of 40–120 mmHg; it usually lasts for 2–4 hours. In this patient, after a meal, there are occasional contractions, but no fed response and the amplitude of phasic contractions is markedly diminished, typical of intestinal myopathy of systemic sclerosis.

131 A 4-year-old child has a history of constipation since infancy. He first passed a meconium stool on day 3 of life. He has always experienced difficulty with bowel movements. Occasionally, when distended, spontaneous, 'explosive', watery bowel movements occur. Currently, he develops severe abdominal distention unless he receives enemas. He has no history of retentive posturing behaviour or soiling. His abdominal radiograph is shown (**131a**).

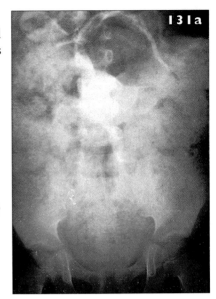

i. What diagnosis should be considered?
ii. What are the possible approaches to diagnostic evaluation?
iii. How is this disorder best treated?
iv. Comment on potential post-treatment complications.

132 Shown (**132**) is an abdominal CT scan after intravenous contrast in a 67-year-old man who presented as an emergency with a 4-hour history of severe upper abdominal pain and mid-back pain. He had a past history of hypertension treated with bendrofluazide 2.5 mg o.d. Examination showed a blood pressure of 95/60 mmHg, and a pulse rate of 105/min. On abdominal examination, a 5 cm liver edge was palpated. The rest of the examination was normal. Investigation results are given in the table.

i. What does the abdominal CT show?
ii. What is the cause of the abdominal pain and hypotension?
iii. What treatment would you institute?

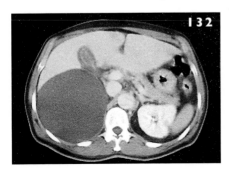

Investigation	Result
Haemoglobin	10.1 g/dl
WBC	$12.6 \times 10^9/l$
Platelets	$423 \times 10^9/l$
U&Es	Normal
Glucose	Normal
Chest radiograph	Normal

131 & 132: Answers

131 i. There is dilatation of the colon. In a 4-year-old, this finding is most commonly observed with functional faecal retentive behaviour. However, this rarely manifests before age 2 years, and associated retentive behaviour and faecal soiling are often present. The delayed passage of meconium and constipation suggests Hirschsprung's disease, characterized by the failure to pass meconium within 24–48 hours of age.

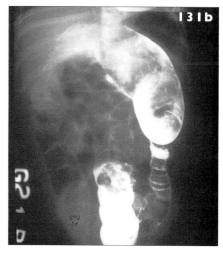

ii. Barium enema usually demonstrates a 'transition zone' from the aganglionic zone to the dilated ganglionated zone (131b). Anorectal manometry demonstrates lack of the anorectal inhibitory reflex. Mucosal suction or full-thickness biopsy with staining for acetylcholinesterase is diagnostic. Histology reveals aganglionosis and mural hypertrophy (131c).

iii. Excision of the aganglionic bowel (131d) with subsequent anal pull-through procedure.

iv. Postoperative enterocolitis develops in 16% of cases. Internal anal sphincterotomy may prevent this occurring.

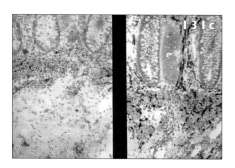
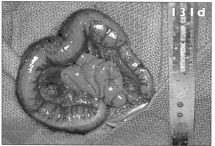

132 i. The abdominal CT (132) shows a large liver cyst which is thin-walled and does not contain contrast.

ii. This is a simple liver cyst; these are usually asymptomatic and do not normally cause complications. The abdominal aorta shows a dissection and further CT scans revealed a thoracic aneurysm extending from the descending aorta.

iii. Treatment consists of supportive management with careful volume replacement and referral for surgery.

133 A 27-year-old woman was investigated for a 2-year history of recurrent abdominal pain and diarrhoea. Her full blood count and colonoscopic findings are shown in the table.
i. What is the diagnosis?
ii. What is the differential diagnosis for the endoscopic appearance (133)?
iii. What treatment options are available?

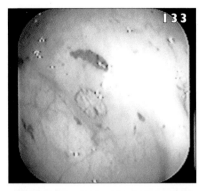

Investigation	Result
Haemoglobin	1.61 mmol/l (10.4 g/dl)
WBC	11.6×10⁹/l
Platelets	577×10⁹/l
ESR	78 mm/h

134 A 27-year-old woman is brought to the emergency room with severe retrosternal pain and odynophagia. She has difficulty handling her secretions and spits into a bowl intermittently. The patient is fully conscious but generally withdrawn. According to her friend, she has a history of depression and previous hospitalizations for suicide attempts, and that morning was found with a half-empty can of drain cleaner next to her bed. She is haemodynamically stable with clear lung fields. The pharynx appears normal. The chest and abdominal radiographs are normal.

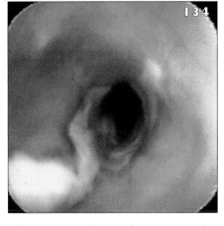

An upper endoscopy, performed during that admission, reveals a narrowed oesophageal lumen with ulcerated overlying mucosa (134).
i. What is the underlying cause of this patient's presenting problem?
ii. Discuss initial (emergency room) management of this patient.
iii. Discuss the determination of the precise extent of the injury.
iv. Review specific medical therapies.
v. Comment on possible long-term complications.

133 i. 133 shows aphthous ulceration. This history and blood picture suggests Crohn's disease.
ii. The differential diagnosis of this appearance includes: amoebiasis; *Herpes simplex* infection; cytomegalovirus infection; Behçet's disease; *Yersinia* infection.
The differential diagnosis is wide and it is imperative that all such lesions are biopsied to make a definitive diagnosis.
iii. Treatment needs to be tailored to the individual patient. The total extent of the disease should be determined. The most useful investigations in addition to colonoscopy are barium enema and barium follow-through (or small-bowel enema). For colonic disease, 5-ASA compounds such as sulphasalazine and mesalamine (mesalazine) are of use both orally and topically. If these are ineffective, antimicrobials or steroids are used.
In small-bowel disease, slow-release 5-ASA compounds have some effect and steroids are useful – as is an elemental diet – although this needs to be strictly adhered to. Immunosuppressives are useful for their steroid-sparing effects. Surgery may eventually become necessary for strictures, fistulas and abscesses.

134 i. This patient has sustained a caustic injury, probably due to lye ingestion. This extremely alkaline substance is capable of causing deep injury.
ii. Identify the type of agent swallowed, and when it was consumed. Some advocate the immediate administration of water or milk to wash the corrosive off the oesophagus. Gastric lavage is contraindicated. Chest and abdominal radiographs may identify mediastinitis, pleural effusions and perforation. Early signs and symptoms are not predictive of the development of oesophageal lesions, and the extent of the injury may be difficult to judge from the oropharyngeal examination.
iii. Inspection of the pharynx and larynx must be performed. Gentle early endoscopy is considered more useful than contrast radiography in determining the extent of the injury in patients who do not have mediastinitis, pleuritis or peritonitis. The injury is staged according to the presence of erythema, ulceration and tissue necrosis.
iv. Nutrition must be maintained. Consideration should be given to a gastrostomy for those with severe burns. There is no uniform agreement regarding the usefulness of a nasogastric tube, and of intravenous corticosteroids and antibiotics with respect to resolution of inflammation or prevention of complications. Sucralfate may confer some benefit. Liquid antacids may alleviate retrosternal discomfort. The development of an oesophageal stricture appears only related to the severity of the corrosive injury.
v. Over 20% of patients develop a stricture (134), the majority of whom require periodic dilatation. Those with impending perforation or intractable strictures require surgery and oesophageal reconstruction. Patients who have sustained an oesophageal lye burn have a 1000-fold greater risk of developing an oesophageal carcinoma 40–60 years after the injury. Periodic surveillance, beginning 20 years after the injury, has been advised. Aorto-oesophageal fistulization may also occur.

135 A 54-year-old warehouseman was referred for evaluation of a 3-month history of intermittent choking sensation, and of dysphagia for solids and more recently for liquids, weight loss and vomiting, which occasionally woke him at night. There was a long-standing history of heartburn that disturbed his sleep. He had become afraid to eat normally for fear of inducing pain and vomiting. He smokes 20 cigarettes per day. He underwent a coronary angioplasty the previous year with good relief of anginal symptoms. He is taking nitrates, calcium channel blockers and H2-receptor antagonists. On examination, he was moderately obese with epigastric tenderness. Haematology and biochemical profiles were normal. A barium study was performed (**135**).

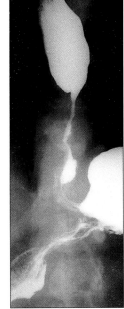

i. What does the history suggest?
ii. Comment on the radiological findings.
iii. What additional investigations may be necessary?
iv. Discuss any pertinent predisposing factors.
v. Comment on treatment modalities applicable for this patient.

136 A 38-year-old man presented with a history of epigastric pain and 4 kg (9 lb) weight loss. A smoker of 40 cigarettes a day, he had found that self-induced vomiting relieved some of his symptoms. Examination was unremarkable. Blood count, urea and electrolytes, and liver function tests were within normal limits. At initial OGD, food residue prevented full assessment. At repeat procedure after a prolonged fast, a malignant-looking gastric ulcer was found. Cytology was unhelpful. *Candida* species were seen in the ulcer slough, but no evidence of malignancy. A CT scan (**136**) of the lower thorax and abdomen was requested.

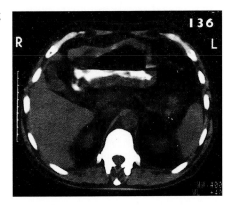

i. What does **136** show?
ii. How should this patient's management proceed?
iii. What is the prognosis?

135 i. The history is strongly suggestive of an oesophageal stricture. The majority are benign and are due to GORD in association with an hiatus hernia. Other common causes include webs; pill-induced, corrosive-induced, post-infective, and post-traumatic strictures, including following radiation to the mediastinum. Motility disorders, as occur in achalasia and scleroderma, may also cause dysphagia. Carcinoma of the oesophagus is a consideration. While the majority of malignancies are squamous lesions, cancers associated with Barrett's oesophagus are adenocarcinomas.

ii. A long symmetrical stricture in the distal oesophagus upstream of a large hiatus hernia is seen.

iii. An upper endoscopy is important to visualize the stricture directly and to sample involved mucosa. Endoscopic ultrasound and CT scanning are sometimes employed when other modalities provide inconclusive results – and for tumour staging. Oesophageal manometry is generally not useful in the work-up of patients with a mechanically significant stricture.

iv. The patient's obesity, lifestyle and occupation may be predisposing factors. In addition, pharmaceutical agents, including calcium-channel and beta-blockers, may further decrease the size of the lower oesophageal sphincter aperture. It is possible that a nasogastric tube, inserted for a prolonged period (the patient underwent surgery the previous year) may have been a complicating factor.

v. Treatment would include oesophageal dilatation, best achieved by an endoscopic technique. Aggressive conservative measures, such as stopping smoking, weight reduction, sleeping with the head-end of the bed elevated, and avoiding tight garments around the waist, are also important. High-dose H2 blockers or proton pump inhibitors are useful in promoting healing and in maintaining remission. Prokinetic agents (cisapride or metoclopramide) may serve as an adjunct to anti-secretory therapy. Surgery is appropriate if symptoms prove refractory. The placement of oesophageal stents is occasionally useful for supportive treatment of malignant lesions that remain symptomatic despite employment of other modalities (surgery, radiotherapy, chemotherapy, laser therapy, etc.).

136 i. The CT scan (**136**) shows a grossly thickened stomach wall and some food residue. The appearances are most in keeping with lymphoma. Multiple biopsies are taken to establish a tissue diagnosis which otherwise may not be known until laparotomy, which may be required to promote gastric emptying.

ii. Primary lymphomas of the stomach represent only 5% of gastric malignancies. They most commonly arise from mucosa-associated lymphoid tissue so are known as MALTomas. Association with *Helicobacter pylori* infection has been proposed and reports exist of resolution of early low-grade tumours with *Helicobacter* eradication therapy. However, standard treatments involve both surgery and radiotherapy.

iii. The prognosis is related to tumour grade and stage. Survival rates approaching 95% at 5 years are not unusual in patients with low-grade disease confined to the stomach.

137 A 67-year-old woman presented with right flank pain radiating to the groin and labia. This responded to an injection of diclofenac with no specific diagnosis being made. After 3 days she represented with similar but more severe pain, now associated with vomiting. She was admitted to hospital. The past history included a superior mesenteric artery thrombosis responsible for infarction of more than 50% of the small intestine, and the infarcted bowel had been resected, leaving an anastomosis between the jejunum and the ascending colon. Underlying atrial fibrillation was implicated and since this episode she had been well on warfarin anticoagulation and a normal diet. There were no physical signs apart from the previous operative scar and localized tenderness in the right-side of the abdomen. Routine laboratory investigations, including full blood count, amylase, and renal and hepatic biochemistry, were normal, but a urine dipstick demonstrated the presence of blood.
i. What is the clinical diagnosis?
ii. What imaging modality is most likely to be helpful?
iii. What, if any, contributory biochemical tests could be run?
iv. What is the likely biochemical diagnosis and its pathogenesis? How can the risk of future episodes be diminished?

138 A 35-year-old immunosuppressed man developed severe abdominal pain shortly after an ERCP performed to investigate obstructive jaundice. During the procedure a biliary stent had been placed across a benign, low, common bile duct stricture attributed to AIDS-related sclerosing cholangitis. A CT scan was obtained (138a) and repeated at 7 days (138b).
i. What is shown in scans 138a and 138b?
ii. What complication is suggested, and how might this be confirmed?
iii. What are the therapeutic options?

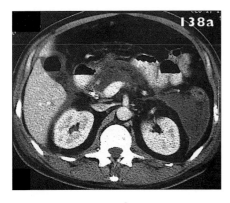
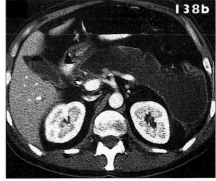

137 i. Right ureteric calculus.
ii. Intravenous urography.
iii. 24-hour urine collection for calcium, oxalate and uric acid.
iv. Calcium oxalate stones.
Within the context of short-bowel syndrome patients, renal calculi occur in almost
one-third, and are usually due to increased absorption of oxalate from the intestine
due to factors which increase the permeability of the colon, e.g. bile salts or fatty
acids, resulting in hyperoxaluria. Intraluminal oxalate is normally bound to calcium
within the small bowel and is not absorbed; if calcium is not available, e.g. due to the
fat malabsorption which occurs after massive small-intestinal resection leaving the fat
to bind to calcium to form soaps, this leaves free oxalate to be absorbed in the colon.
Calcium then binds with oxalate in the urine. Generally, this applies to those with a
short gut anastomosed to the colon, and patients with a jejunostomy are not prone to
oxalate stones. Risk of future episodes may be diminished by:
• Dietary oxalate restriction, e.g. spinach, rhubarb, parsley, cocoa, beetroot, tea,
  peppers, peanuts, chocolate. On a daily basis tea is the most important source.
• Oral calcium supplements – these help to precipitate oxalates in the intestinal
  lumen.
• Cholestyramine – this binds to fatty acids, bile acids and oxalate in the colon.
• Oral citrate – to enhance urine solubility of oxalate.

138 i. 138a shows a swollen and necrotic pancreas with an adjacent collection of
fluid alongside the tail. 138b shows almost complete liquefaction of the pancreas and
a resultant large intra-abdominal fluid collection.
ii. This indicates severe necrotizing pancreatitis, a diagnosis supported by finding a
high serum amylase and lipase in conjunction with hypocalcaemia and
electrolyte/acid–base disturbance. Had doubt existed, a diagnostic tap of the fluid
collection and amylase estimation of its content would have been helpful, albeit with
a finite risk of precipitating infection. Acute pancreatitis is a recognized complication
of ERCP. Mild and transient elevation of pancreatic enzymes is common and
clinically apparent pancreatitis occurs in at least 1% of patients. Severe pancreatitis
should be rare with appropriate attention to cannula sterility and endoscope
cleansing protocols, but still affects up to 0.03% of diagnostic cases and nearly 1%
when a sphincterotomy has been performed. It is more likely when the procedure has
been difficult or lengthy, or when over-filling of the pancreatic duct and thereby
filling of the parenchyma has occurred.
iii. Mild cases of acute ERCP-related pancreatitis settle with conservative
management comprising intravenous fluid, bowel rest and analgesia. Severe
necrotizing pancreatitis has a high morbidity and mortality. Haemodynamic and
renal support may be required. Antibiotics are then mandatory. Metabolic and
coagulation defects should be corrected, with consideration of surgical debridement
of necrotic tissue.

139 A 70-year-old widow presented with a 6-month history of postprandial epigastric pain and anorexia. Her weight was steady. She was on regular vitamin B_{12} for pernicious anaemia and thyroxine for myxoedema. She smoked, but avoided alcohol. Some 21 years earlier she had had surgery for duodenal ulcer disease: first a vagotomy and pyloroplasty; then a Billroth I partial gastrectomy a year later.

Examination revealed vitiligo but was otherwise normal. Routine laboratory tests were also normal. **139** shows the appearance at endoscopy (before biopsy).

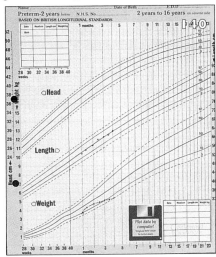

i. What is shown and what risk factors are exemplified?
ii. What further investigations are indicated, if any?
iii. How should further management be determined and what is the prognosis?

140 A 16-week-old male presented with diarrhoea and failure to thrive. He was born to non-consanguineous parents, both well. He had been breast-fed since birth. At 8 weeks he was admitted with pyrexia, bloodless diarrhoea and respiratory distress. A diagnosis of right lower lobe pneumonia was made and successfully treated with antibiotics including clarithromycin. After discharge the child began vomiting and had explosive diarrhoea with occasional blood in the stools. He became very miserable and had screaming episodes at night with poor feeding and failure to thrive. Full blood count and urea and electrolytes were normal. The serum albumin was 27 g/l; faecal occult blood was positive. **140** shows the growth chart.

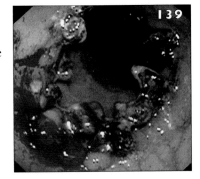

On admission, breast feeding was stopped, oral rehydration solution was given, and in 24 hours the diarrhoea ceased. Breast feeding was recommenced and the diarrhoea recurred.

i. What are the most likely diagnoses?
ii. What investigations are called for?

139 & 140: Answers

139 i. Gastric carcinoma at the anastomosis (139). Risk factors include prior partial gastrectomy and pernicious anaemia. There is a positive association with nitrates in food preservation, and with pickled and salted foods. Refrigeration may contribute to the falling incidence. This contrasts with a rising incidence of carcinoma of the distal oesophagus and cardia. *Helicobacter pylori* infection is associated with gastric cancer. This may follow from the development of atrophic gastritis and intestinal metaplasia. Adenomatous polyps are also premalignant. Familial clustering occurs and there is a positive association with blood group A.
ii. Biopsy is essential to confirm the diagnosis. Metastases are sought by chest radiography and liver imaging.
iii. Management depends on the presence or absence of extragastric spread. Staging, assisted by endoscopic ultrasound, may help determine whether surgery can be contemplated with curative or palliative intent. Levels of tumour markers have little role. Disease confined to the mucosa has a 5-year survival rate over 90%, but once the serosa is breached fewer than 10% of patients survive 5 years. Unfortunately, most have unresectable disease. The overall median survival is 15 months. Only in Asian centres (a high rate of early gastric carcinoma) do better results emerge. Surgery offers the best palliation in a patient in whom the general state appears good, especially when there are obstructive features present. Radiotherapy does not have a major role, but chemotherapy can add usefully to survival.

140 i. Cows' milk-sensitive enteropathy (CMSE) with or without lactose intolerance. Cystic fibrosis or pseudomembranous colitis are also possible. Lactose intolerance alone and cystic fibrosis are unlikely because of the presence of bleeding. Pseudomembranous colitis is unlikely because in this disorder the diarrhoea continues despite fasting.
CMSE is characterized by a mucosal reaction to the proteins in cow's milk. Patchy partial villous atrophy is seen. CMSE can occur in breast-fed infants because of the transmission of cow's milk proteins via maternal milk. It may occur following gastroenteritis or without any obvious precipitating event, in which case failure to thrive may be the only feature. Lactose malabsorption occurs if there is significant loss of microvillous lactase activity. This is characterized by the presence of reducing substances in an acid stool (pH <5.5); cows' milk should be eliminated from the diet. If breast feeding is continued, the mother should eliminate cows' milk from her diet. If she discontinues breast feeding, a commercial cows' milk-free formula should be used. Unfortunately, 30–50% of infants also react to soya proteins, so hydrolysate formulations are best used. CMSE has a variable duration and may extend from 3 months to 2 years.
ii. Tests for the presence of reducing substances, pH, and *Clostridium difficile* toxin in the stool. A small-bowel biopsy and sweat test should be considered.

141 A 48-year-old man with ulcerative
colitis presents with a relapse of his disease.
In addition, over the past few weeks he has
developed a marked abnormality of the skin
(141). It is not painful nor pruritic. He is not
taking any medications.
i. What is this skin lesion?
ii. Comment on its histology and its
relationship to bowel disease activity.
iii. What treatment options are available for
this lesion related to inflammatory bowel
disease?
iv. Comment on other dermatological
manifestations of inflammatory bowel
disease.

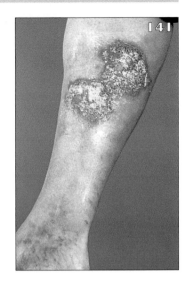

142 A 23-year-old college senior on a
gymnastics scholarship complains to
her team physician of fatigue and
painful 'leg bumps' (142). She has had
two or three loose, non-bloody bowel
movements daily over the past 3
months and a 4.5 kg (10 lb) weight loss.
She exercises for about 3 hours each
day, eats meals with the gymnastics

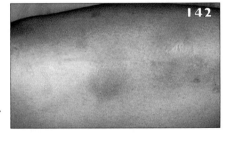

team and takes numerous multi-vitamin supplements, an over-the-counter
protein supplement and three over-the-counter zinc tablets a day to improve
her endurance. Her menstrual history is unremarkable. Routine blood
screening revealed a haemoglobin of 9.8 g/dl; haematocrit of 29%; MCV of
80 fl; and neutropenia.
i. What is the dermatological diagnosis?
ii. What are the disease processes associated with these lesions?
iii. Comment on the haematological abnormalities.
iv. A bone marrow examination demonstrates normal iron stores, and the
serum copper and caeruloplasmin levels were both significantly decreased.
How may this be related to the above history?
v. What are the manifestations of copper deficiency and how should this
patient be treated?

141 i. The two most common dermatological extraintestinal manifestations of inflammatory bowel disease are erythema nodosum and, as in this patient, pyoderma gangrenosum (PG).
ii. These lesions are vasculitic in nature and often parallel disease activity in the bowel. However, presentation may antedate that of the bowel component, or indeed occur for the first time following colectomy.
iii. Typical therapy for inflammatory bowel disease, with corticosteroids and mesalamine (mesalazine), often successfully treats pyoderma. Resistant cases require more intense immunosuppression with azathioprine, 6-mercaptopurine, cyclosporin or dapsone. Oral broad-spectrum antibiotics to control superinfection are helpful and topical steroids may reduce induration and erythema at the margin of the lesions. For extremely severe pyoderma refractory to therapy, surgical resection of the colon and, less often, of the area of active inflammation, is indicated.
iv. Other, less common dermatological manifestations of inflammatory bowel disease include psoriasis, aphthous stomatitis, 'metastatic' Crohn's disease of the skin, epidermolysis bullosa acquisita, and neutrophilic dermatosis (Sweet's syndrome).

142 i. The skin lesions over the leg are erythema nodosum.
ii. Many systemic disease processes are associated with erythema nodosum, including Crohn's disease; infectious processes such as tuberculosis, histoplasmosis, coccidioidomycosis, and streptococcal infection; sarcoidosis; ulcerative colitis; and drugs such as penicillin, and sulphonamides, and certain oral contraceptives. In this girl, a colonoscopy showed typical lesions of Crohn's disease in the caecum and the terminal ileum.
iii. Likely causes of this patient's anaemia are iron deficiency due to poor absorption (resulting from Crohn's disease or an additional intestinal problem such as coeliac disease), poor intake due to dieting (an unusual cause of iron deficiency in developed countries), intestinal loss due to inflammatory bowel disease (although the patient has not observed any overt bleeding), or menstrual loss (but the patient denies excessive bleeding). Iron deficiency, however, is not associated with neutropenia. Other causes of microcytosis include thalassaemia, sideroblastic anaemia and copper deficiency.
iv. Thus, this patient likely has a copper-deficiency anaemia and neutropenia. The patient could be copper-deficient due to copper malabsorption as a result of her Crohn's disease, or from zinc–copper interactions due to her over-the-counter zinc supplementation. The most likely cause of the patient's copper deficiency is zinc supplementation. Zinc and copper interact at the intestinal level. High doses of zinc induce production of the metal-binding protein, metallothionein, the natural regulatory mechanism for zinc and copper absorption. The high-dose zinc supplementation impairs copper absorption and ultimately causes copper deficiency, the rationale for using zinc supplementation in the treatment of Wilson's disease.
v. Clinical manifestations of copper deficiency include hypochromic microcytic anaemia, leukopenia, neutropenia and scurvy-like skeletal abnormalities. The patient can be treated by discontinuing zinc supplementation and possibly by giving low-dose copper supplementation (1–2 mg copper/day).

143 A 46-year-old man, an unrestrained passenger in a motor vehicle accident, was admitted with a Glasgow Coma Scale Score of 4, together with severe head trauma and cerebral oedema. Parenteral nutrition was initiated shortly after admission. The levels of prealbumin and albumin, and protein intake, are shown (143).

i. Why were the albumin and prealbumin levels initially low?

ii. What are the approximate half-lives of the four visceral proteins frequently used as indicators of nutritional status (albumin, transferrin, prealbumin, retinol binding protein) and why might the half-life of such a protein be important?

iii. Does the continually decreasing serum albumin level in this patient necessarily indicate that he requires more nitrogen in his intravenous feed?

iv. Why might the serum albumin still be declining in this patient?

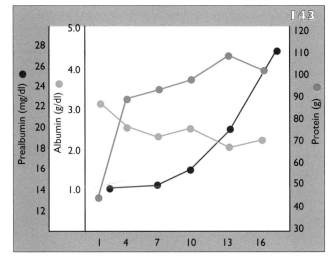

144 A 72-year-old man presented with a 2-month history of vomiting within a few hours of eating. He had lost 19 kg (42 lb) in weight during this time. He was clinically anaemic, and there was epigastric fullness and an equivocal succussion splash on examination (144).

i. What is shown?

ii. Discuss the proposed aetiological factors for this condition.

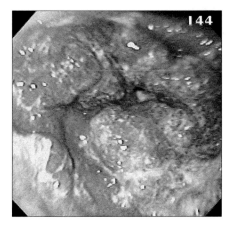

143 i. Following any kind of major trauma there is an increased vascular leak with loss of proteins such as albumin and prealbumin.

ii. Half-lives are 18–21 days, 8 days, 2 days and 0.5 days, respectively. The more rapid turnover proteins such as prealbumin are an earlier indicator of nutritional status.

iii. Overall protein intake and nitrogen balance are critical issues. The patient was shown to be taking in adequate amounts and was in positive nitrogen balance. Thus, the nitrogen balance is more critical than visceral protein levels in assessing nitrogen needs.

iv. The serum albumin may still be decreasing because of the patient's overall critically ill status. The inflammatory cytokines such as IL-1 and TNF down-regulate mRNA for albumin production. Moreover, there could be continued vascular leak of albumin. Thus, the albumin and other visceral proteins really reflect overall clinical status and not necessarily just nutritional status. The fact that the prealbumin is responding more quickly relates, at least in part, to its shorter half-life.

144 i. 144 shows an irregular lesion around the pylorus, causing an outflow obstruction. Histology confirmed a gastric adenocarcinoma.

ii. The aetiology is due to the interaction of a large number of factors.

The incidence varies from country to country. Japan has a very high incidence, previously felt to be due to a high salt intake, but some countries with a higher per capita salt intake have a lower incidence. Since refrigerators have become commonplace the incidence has decreased, perhaps due to reduction in the formation of carcinogens produced by alternative forms of preservation.

Those people with a high intake of N-nitroso compounds are more at risk. These compounds are strongly carcinogenic and are formed spontaneously in the stomach from amines in certain foods. Such formation preferentially occurs at neutral pH. Thus, those people with low acid production/achlorhydria produce more N-nitroso compounds. However, to date, acid suppression with proton pump inhibitors has not been associated with the development of gastric neoplasia.

H. pylori, by inducing chronic gastritis, may lead to tumorigenesis.

Alcohol has not been implicated in the formation of cancer, although smoking may be. There is also some evidence of a genetic predisposition and the expression of the p53 protein is associated with an increased risk of gastric cancer and poorer prognosis.

145 A 65-year-old man has a 6-month history of change in bowel habit with episodes of small-volume haematochezia. A flexible sigmoidoscopy demonstrates a 4 cm mass lesion at 40 cm (145a). It is firm to probing with the biopsy forceps.
i. What is the likely diagnosis?
ii. What further information would be helpful in treatment planning?
iii. What is the appropriate treatment?
iv. Comment on the molecular basis for this lesion, and on the role of screening for this lesion in asymptomatic individuals.

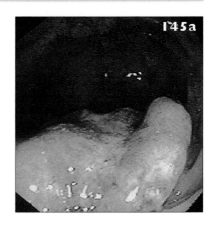

146 A 48-year-old man has long-standing heartburn with occasional nocturnal vomiting. An oesophagogram in the past demonstrated moderately severe reflux. He has gained weight over the years, and his symptoms continue despite H2-receptor antagonist therapy. An upper endoscopy reveals reflux of gastric contents into the oesophagus (146a) and gastric mucosa extending 5 cm into the distal tubular oesophagus (146b).
i. What is the diagnosis?
ii. How can this be confirmed?
iii. Describe management strategies for the underlying condition.
iv. Discuss strategies aimed at reversing the lesion.
v. Discuss complications and their prevention.

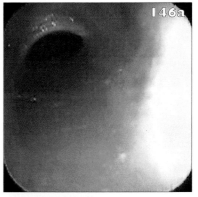

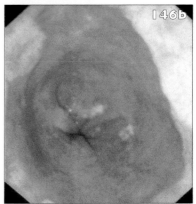

145 & 146: Answers

145 i. Colon carcinoma.
ii. Synchronous cancers are found at presentation in approximately 4% of cases; therefore, the entire colon is visualized before surgery. 145b demonstrates an 'apple-core' lesion. A CT scan of the abdomen may facilitate staging. CEA levels are often employed to monitor for possible preclinical recurrence following resection.
iii. Resection, the approach and extent depending on the vascular supply and the

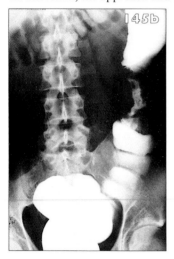

tumour-free margins. Lymph node involvement is an indication for adjuvant chemotherapy.
iv. A series of mutations must occur for colonic mucosa to become adenomatous, to develop cytologic atypia and finally frank carcinoma. One potential initial mutation occurs in the *APC* gene. In sporadic colorectal cancer the mutation is somatic (i.e. limited to the polyp itself), while in familial adenomatous polyposis, the mutation is germline and passed in an autosomal dominant fashion. Annual faecal occult blood testing reduces colorectal cancer mortality by 33%. Periodic screening sigmoidoscopy (5-yearly) has been demonstrated to have a favourable impact on mortality from colon cancer.

146 i. GORD with Barrett's oesophagus.
ii. The normal (white) squamous epithelium of the distal tubular oesophagus is replaced by an epithelium with features of both gastric and intestinal mucosae. Biopsies most commonly demonstrate specialized columnar epithelium, an incomplete form of intestinal metaplasia. Other types include junctional-type and gastric fundic-type epithelium. Barrett's oesophagus develops as a complication in 10% of patients with chronic GORD.
iii. Management includes raising the head of the bed, weight reduction, antisecretory therapy with proton pump blockers and prokinetic agents. Surgery may be necessary for intractable symptoms.
iv. Neither medical nor surgical measures reverse Barrett's epithelium. Photodynamic therapy is currently being utilized in selective situations in an attempt to re-epithelialize Barrett's oesophagus with squamous epithelium.
v. Patients with Barrett's are prone to all the complications of GORD. About 5% of patients with Barrett's develop an oesophageal adenocarcinoma. Barrett's oesophagus therefore has neoplastic potential. Periodic endoscopic surveillance employing multiple biopsies is advocated for the detection of dysplastic changes or the diagnosis of carcinoma at an early stage. Resection is reserved for those patients with established cancer and confirmed high-grade dysplasia. Treatment of those with low-grade dysplasia must be individualized.

147 Answer TRUE or FALSE regarding octreotide (somatostatin analogue) being beneficial in the following situations:
i. Oesophageal variceal haemorrhage.
ii. Acute pancreatitis.
iii. Chronic pancreatitis.
iv. VIPoma.
v. Actively bleeding peptic ulcer.

148 A 16-year-old boy is referred by his school doctor because of recurrent time off from school with abdominal pain. Having previously performed well at school, his performance in the past 2 years has deteriorated. Furthermore, he lost 5 kg (11 lb) in weight in the preceding year and produced loose stool. He also describes severe pain in his large joints and has been unable to play games at school for 6 months. Examination reveals a slight boy with pale skin and no lymphadenopathy or fever, and that his joints are normal but there is pain on palpation of his rib cage and spine. He has glossitis and oral mucosal ulcers. He has scant pubic hair and small testes. His abdomen is distended with generalized abdominal pain. There is no ascites. Rectal examination is normal with normal stool on glove. Investigation results are are given in the table.

148a shows the endoscopic appearances in the proximal duodenum after indigo carmine dye application to the mucosal surface.

Investigation	Result
Haemoglobin	12.1 g/dl
MCV	72 fl
WBC	4.1×10^9/l
Platelets	412×10^9/l
U&Es	Normal
Bilirubin	12 µmol/l (0.7 mg/dl)
SGPT	16 u/l (normal 15–30 u/l)
ALP	468 u/l (normal 150–300 u/l)
Albumin	33 g/l
Calcium	2.02 mmol/l (8.1 mg/dl)
RA latex	Negative

i. What is the likely diagnosis?
ii. What other investigations are needed to support the diagnosis?
iii. Discuss the bone and joint symptoms.
iv. What are the key points in advising the parents on management?
v. If the patient fails to respond initially, what are the possible explanations?

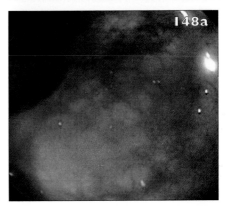
148a

147 & 148: Answers

147 i. True. Octreotide decreases splanchnic and portal blood flow and has been shown to be efficacious for haemostasis in patients with variceal haemorrhage – comparable with balloon tamponade and vasopressin plus nitroglycerin with a significantly lower incidence of complications.

ii. True. Meta-analysis demonstrates a significant decrease in the mortality and morbidity of patients with severe acute pancreatitis treated with octreotide.

iii. False. A clear benefit has not been demonstrated.

iv. True. Somatostatin reduces diarrhoea in patients with carcinoid syndrome and VIPomas.

v. False. Studies indicate no significant effect.

148 i. Coeliac disease. The mucosa shows a flat pattern compared with the normal appearance in **148b**. The abnormality comprises crypt elongation opening onto a flat

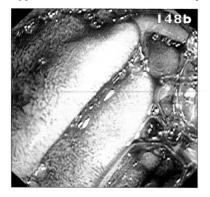

absorptive surface with absent or shrunken villi, along with increased cellularity in the lamina propria. A gluten-free diet normalizes mucosal architecture. These abnormalities are also seen in lactose intolerance, giardiasis and Zollinger–Ellison syndrome.

ii. Confirmatory investigations include:
- Jejunal biopsy, repeated after abstinence from gluten-containing products for 12 weeks.
- Anti-endomysium, anti-reticulin and anti-gliadin antibodies.
- Malabsorption profile and growth chart plotting are also useful.

iii. The bone pain and tenderness is probably consequent upon osteopaenic bone disease (calcium and vitamin D malabsorption) as evidenced by hypocalcaemia and raised ALP. Radiography of the joints may show typical changes (demineralization, milkman's lines and vertebral compression fractures) and provide an estimate of bone age.

iv. Life-long dietary modification needs to be discussed with patient, parents and a dietician. Milk products should be consumed in moderation initially (higher incidence of secondary lactase deficiency).

Realistic expectations of height 'catching-up' are given. The need for occasional review should be emphasized – to monitor for associated diseases (dermatitis herpetiformis, arthritis, type I diabetes, non-specific colitis) and the rare complications of coeliac disease, namely small-intestinal stricture or ulceration, refractory sprue or intestinal malignancy.

v. Mis-diagnosis; poor adherence to diet; refractory or collagenous sprue; small-intestinal lymphoma.

The prognosis for coeliac disease, once the diagnosis has been established is very good, with normal life expectancy – most deaths result from unrelated conditions. Untreated, it may be fatal.

149 A 30-year-old woman with type I diabetes mellitus presents with a 3-year history of episodic projectile vomiting, which has led to multiple admissions with diabetic ketoacidosis. She also reports constipation since childhood, with a stool frequency of once a week. Medications include insulin, enemas and half a gallon of polyethylene glycol solution every third day. On examination she is comfortable, and has palpable stool in both lower quadrants. Bowel sounds are normal. Rectal examination reveals copious, firm stool. Tests demonstrate normal haemoglobin, white cell count, liver enzymes, lipase, urea and electrolytes. The blood glucose is 11.1 mmol/l (200 mg/dl), haemoglobin A_{1C} 9%. A solid phase gastric emptying scan is shown in **149a**, colonic transit marker study in **149b**, and anorectal manometry in **149c**.
i. On the basis of the history, which disorders should be considered?
ii. Which investigations are appropriate?
iii. Comment on **149a**.
iv. Comment on the radiograph shown in **149b**.
v. Comment on the anorectal manometry tracings shown in **149c**.
vi. What is the diagnosis and appropriate treatment?

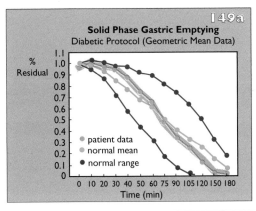

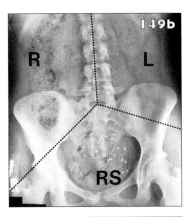

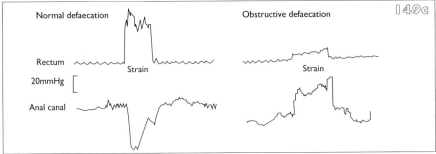

149: Answers

149 i. The differential diagnosis includes: (a) diabetic ketoacidosis with brittle diabetes; (b) gastric outlet obstruction; (c) gastroparesis; (d) chronic constipation; and (e) intestinal obstruction.

ii. Investigations should include biochemical, electrolyte and thyroid profiles to exclude a metabolic disturbance. An erect radiograph of the abdomen may reveal excess stool or bowel obstruction. Endoscopy or barium meal with follow-through may demonstrate gastric outlet disease or obstruction. A gastric emptying study may reveal gastroparesis. Colonic obstruction is demonstrated by colonoscopy or enema. A colon transit marker study identifies slow transit constipation (colonic inertia). Anorectal manometry may reveal pelvic floor dysfunction.

iii. The scintigraphic gastric emptying test consists of administering a radioisotope bound to either scrambled eggs or chicken liver, and serial scanning is then performed. The amount of residual gastric radiotracer is plotted. 149a shows the mean gastric emptying time with 95% confidence intervals for normal subjects. The patient's profile (orange line in broad grey band) demonstrates normal emptying, excluding gastroparesis.

iv. 149b shows a supine radiograph of the abdomen performed 120 hours after ingestion of a capsule containing radio-opaque markers, utilized to evaluate colon transit time. The patient refrains from using laxatives, suppositories or enemas and eats normally for the 5 days following ingestion of the capsule. The number of markers remaining in each zone (149b) are counted; normally there are five or less remaining. Markers distributed throughout the colon indicate slow transit constipation or colonic inertia. If confined to the rectosigmoid region, a diagnosis of obstructive defecation is substantiated.

v. When asked to bear down as if to defaecate, a normal subject shows a rise in intrarectal pressure associated with relaxation of the anal canal. This patient shows a minimal increase in rectal pressure and a paradoxical increase in anal pressure (149c), which are characteristic of obstructive defaecation (anismus, pelvic floor dyssynergia, outlet obstruction). In this disorder, the subject inadvertently closes the anal canal instead of relaxing during defaecation. It affects 30–50% of patients with chronic constipation.

vi. This patient has obstructive defaecation with constipation and functional intestinal obstruction. Optimal treatment consists in retraining using neuromuscular conditioning and biofeedback techniques, in conjunction with enhanced fluid and fibre intake, exercise, saline laxatives and habit retraining.

150 A 26-year-old woman presented
after a holiday in Kenya, where she
had developed diarrhoea, with some
blood and mucus and a slight fever. She
had not previously sought medical
advice for two previous milder episodes.
She had received all the appropriate
vaccines before her holiday and had
taken the recommended malarial
prophylaxis, but probably had
unprotected sexual intercourse with a man she met on holiday. Initial
investigations were unhelpful, so colonoscopy was performed (150).
i. What abnormalities are shown?
ii. What is the differential diagnosis?

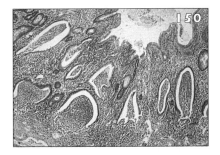

151 A 50-year-old man has a history of progressive watery diarrhoea that has
increased dramatically in the past 3 months. He has not travelled to any
developing countries in the past 2 years. He describes the diarrhoea as
watery, with the appearance of 'weak tea', but never bloody. He was briefly
admitted to hospital 2 months previously for intravenous volume
replacement. Stool specimens for WBCs, culture, and ova and parasites were
all negative. A flexible sigmoidoscopy with random biopsies in the sigmoid
and rectum was normal. He now presents to the emergency room with
fatigue and weakness from persistent diarrhoea. He is markedly dehydrated
with a serum sodium of 130 mmol/l (normal, 133–143 mmol/l), potassium
1.6 mmol/l (normal, 3.5–5.3 mmol/l), BUN 20 mmol/l (28 mg/dl) [normal
7.1–14.1 mmol/l (10–20 mg/dl)] and a creatinine of 106 µmol/l (1.2 mg/dl)
[normal, 53–88 µmol/l (0.6–1.0 mg/dl)]. Fasting serum gastrin is 76 pg/ml. A
stool laxative screen is negative. Laboratory data obtained on this admission
are given in the table.
i. How do you interpret these laboratory data?
ii. Are any other
biochemical studies
indicated?
iii. Should an abdominal CT
scan or other imaging study
be ordered?
iv. How should the
diarrhoea be managed?

Test	Stools (admission)	Stools (fasting)	NG suction
Volume (l/24 h)	6	5.3	5.4
Sodium (mmol/l)	95	125	105
Potassium (mmol/l)	50	30	45
Osmolarity (mosmol/l)	304	330	325

150 i. The colonoscopic appearances were felt most likely to be those of ulcerative colitis and this was supported by the histology of the biopsies which not only showed evidence of an acute colitis, with crypt abscesses and goblet cell depletion, but also the architectural changes of the crypts typical of chronic disease. 'Hot' stools were negative for pathogens and sexually transmitted diseases were not found.
ii. The differential diagnosis includes infective diarrhoea – which should include sexually transmitted organisms such as gonorrhoea – and idiopathic inflammatory bowel disease. There are no other likely diagnoses but it would be wise to exclude malaria given the patient's temperature.

151 i. These data are typical of a severe secretory diarrhoea. The stool osmolar gap, measured as stool osmolarity minus 2(stool $\{[Na^+]+[K^+]\}$) is <50 mosmol/l, suggesting that no additional osmotically active substances are present. The stool osmolarity is within the normal range (275–350 mosmol/l), similar to that of serum. Secretory diarrhoea classically persists in the presence of fasting.
ii. Long-standing, high-volume secretory diarrhoea in such a patient is likely due to the VIPoma syndrome, Zollinger–Ellison syndrome (ZES) or laxative abuse. Factitious diarrhoea characterized by an osmolarity that is higher than expected suggests contamination with urine, whereas one that is lower than expected suggests contamination with water. The negative laxative screen and the absence of unmeasured cations (i.e. an osmolar gap) effectively rules out this possibility. The secretory diarrhoea of ZES classically responds to nasogastric suction since it is entirely due to acid hypersecretion. However, the serum gastrin is normal. In the VIPoma syndrome, diarrhoea is due to autonomous secretion of VIP from a neuroendocrine tumour. Serum VIP levels are elevated during periods when the patient is experiencing diarrhoea. No reliable provocative test is currently available.
iii. VIPomas are usually solitary tumours of the pancreas (98% of cases). Most are >3 cm at presentation and are readily localized by imaging. An octreoscan may also be useful in localization of a suspected neuroendocrine tumour.
iv. Octreotide is indicated for managing a symptomatic VIPoma. VIPomas are commonly malignant and many are metastatic at presentation. In the absence of obvious metastases surgical cure is attempted.

152 Shown (152) is a meglumine
diatrizoate enema in a boy aged 16 years
with a lifelong history of constipation and
faecal soiling.
i. What is the most likely diagnosis?
ii. How should the condition be
managed?

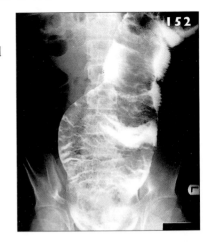

153 A 49-year-old woman presents
with generalized weakness and easy
fatiguability for 6 months, recent
onset of paraesthesia and numbness
in her legs. She is found to have a
macrocytic anaemia (153a) with a
low serum vitamin B_{12} level. An
upper endoscopy reveals a number of
polypoid lesions in the proximal
stomach (153b) which are biopsied.
A Schilling's test is performed.
i. What additional tests may be useful
to work up the cause of the anaemia?
ii. Describe the abnormalities present
on the blood smear in 153a, and the
probable nature of the gastric lesions.
iii. If her stage I Schilling's test for
vitamin B_{12} absorption is normal,
what is the differential diagnosis for
the deficiency?
iv. If the stage I Schilling's test is
abnormal but corrects with intrinsic
factor (IF), what is the diagnosis?
v. If the stage I Schilling's test is
abnormal but does not correct with IF, what is the diagnosis?
vi. Describe management of this patient.

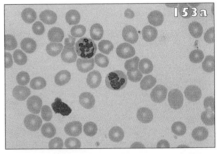

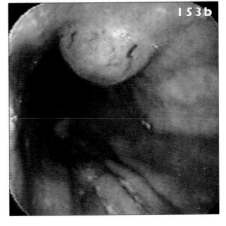

152 i. Idiopathic megarectum with megacolon is most likely (152).
ii. Regular use of laxatives and enemas is the preferred therapy, but subtotal colectomy may be needed. The presence of soiling makes Hirschsprung's disease less likely. The dilatation of the rectum down to the anal canal, without a preserved narrow transitional zone, also argues strongly against Hirschsprung's. Rectal biopsy is hardly necessary.

There appears to be more of a problem with impaired rectal elasticity than with impaired sensation in megarectum patients, although with prolonged untreated disease the normal inhibitory rectoanal reflex may be lost. Symptoms may develop in early childhood or not until early adulthood. Males present much earlier on average.

153 i. The findings are suggestive of pernicious anaemia (PA). Gastric biopsy demonstrates type A (autoimmune) gastritis in the gastric body with paucity of parietal cells, and a gastric juice pH of >4.0. Antral G-cells hypertrophy to produce an elevated serum gastrin. A Schilling's test and parietal cell antibodies may be confirmatory.
ii. Macrocytosis and hypersegmentation of polymorphonuclear leukocytes. PA is a risk factor for gastric adenocarcinoma. However, chronic hypergastrinaemic states are associated with endocrine cell hyperplasia and gastric carcinoids. Although the majority are benign, metastatic disease may occur. These lesions were carcinoids.
iii. The stage I Schilling's is performed by administering radiolabelled B_{12} orally following intramuscular unlabelled vitamin B_{12}. Since the unlabelled vitamin B_{12} saturates all receptor sites, any of the labelled vitamin B_{12} absorbed from the intestine is excreted in the urine. A normal test indicates IF availability. Deficiencies in this setting include poor dietary intake and hypochlorhydria – as acid is required to free dietary B_{12} bound to protein.
iv. In PA, stage I Schilling's is corrected by administration of IF. Antibodies directed against parietal cells that secrete both acid and IF lead to achlorhydria and absent IF.
v. If the stage I Schilling's is not corrected by IF, the patient could still have PA. As many as 30% of cases may not correct, as the disease may alter the receptors in the terminal ileum rendering the vitamin B_{12}–IF complex not able to bind. Causes of 'non correction' include pancreatic insufficiency, bacterial overgrowth, and diseased or absent terminal ileum.
vi. She will require lifelong vitamin B_{12} therapy. Metastatic carcinoids should be excluded by CT scan and 24-hour urinary 5-HIAA collection. The risk of malignancy increases with increasing tumour size. Lesions >2cm are removed. Endoscopic ultrasound assessment may be useful to determine whether they are amenable to endoscopic removal. Opinion is divided as to whether an antrectomy, to eliminate gastrin stimulation, should be performed.

154 A 32-year-old woman is referred for evaluation of chronic abdominal pain which occurs 3–4 times per month, lasts 1–2 days, and is associated with watery bowel movements. Following the bowel movement the pain improves. In between episodes the bowel movements are completely normal. The pain is more likely to occur during times of stress. The discomfort is worse during menstruation. She denies weight loss, blood in the stool, and nocturnal symptoms. The patient's mother experienced similar symptoms when young, but no other family history is of note. Physical examination shows a woman of healthy appearance with increased bowel sounds and a negative test for occult blood. During the past 6 months the patient has had a negative ova and parasite evaluation, a negative sigmoidoscopy with biopsy, a negative barium enema and a normal blood count and ESR. The 24-hour stool weight was 180 g.
i. What is the most likely diagnosis?
ii. Discuss the pathophysiology of this condition.
iii. What further diagnostic tests are needed to confirm the diagnosis?
iv. What treatment would you start at this time?
v. Comment on prognosis.

155 A 64-year-old man is admitted to hospital with abdominal cramps, diarrhoea and dehydration. There is no haematochezia. He has moderate chronic obstructive pulmonary disease and recently developed bronchitis for which he took cefuroxime for 7 days. He has mild abdominal distention and diffuse tenderness. Laboratory investigations reveal: haemoglobin 11.4 g/dl; white cell count 13.9×10^9/l (13900/mm³); and moderate faecal leukocytes (**155a**). A flexible sigmoidoscopy reveals abnormal mucosa (**155b**).

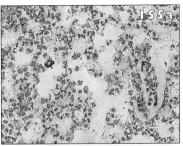
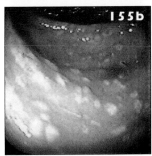

i. Comment on the sigmoidoscopic appearances.
ii. What is the diagnosis?
iii. How may the diagnosis be confirmed?
iv. How is this condition best treated?
v. Comment on possible complications of this disorder.

154 & 155: Answers

154 i. The chronicity of symptoms in the setting of good health, relationship to stress and absence of nocturnal symptomatology suggests irritable bowel syndrome.
ii. This disorder is probably a heterogeneous one, including disordered bowel motility and altered visceral sensation. A history of sexual abuse may be present. Depression is common.
iii. Because the data do not suggest a structural disorder, further testing is unnecessary.
iv. Reassurance and symptomatic treatment of any diarrhoea, constipation or cramping (anticholinergic). An antidepressant might be beneficial.
v. Strategies aimed at control of symptoms and precipitating events are useful.

155 i. 155a shows the classic adherent yellow-white plaques of PMC.
ii. *Clostridium difficile* colitis occurs when the normal bowel flora is altered (usually by antibiotics with activity against anaerobes), followed by nosocomial colonization, and growth of *C. difficile* with toxin elaboration.
iii. Stool assays for *C. difficile* toxin. Sigmoidoscopy with biopsy of abnormal-appearing mucosa. The pseudomembrane is composed of exudate (155c) which appears to erupt from the site of epithelial necrosis. The bowel may become very oedematous (155d) producing 'thumbprinting' radiologically.
iv. Metronidazole is as effective as oral vancomycin, less expensive, and may be given orally or intravenously. Vancomycin must be given orally. Bacitracin is not as effective. Cholestyramine binds the toxin but has no effect on the bacterium. Manoeuvres to alter the bacterial flora in an attempt to reconstitute the intraluminal microbiological environment – including the use of *Lactobacillus* and *Saccharomyces boulardii* – have been attempted.
v. Toxic megacolon and perforation may occur. Relapse rates are in excess of 15%. Persistence of spores may play a role, and may require a prolonged course of intermittent therapy.

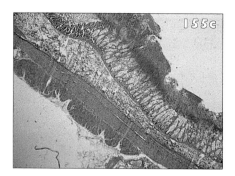
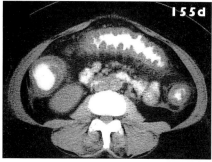

156 A 43-year-old man presented to the emergency service with a large haematemesis. The appearance at upper GI endoscopy is shown (156).
i. What is the lesion?
ii. How else may such a lesion present?

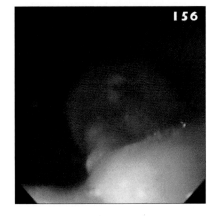

157 A 62-year-old woman was referred because of heartburn and dysphagia, which was maximal when eating bread. An initial response to antacids had been lost over the 6 months before referral this effect. There was a past history of mastectomy for breast cancer and she was still on tamoxifen. She smoked daily and drank a bottle of sherry every other day. 157a shows the initial endoscopic appearance of the gastro-oesophageal junction; 157b shows the junction again 3 years later after increasing dysphagia and 5 kg (11 lb) weight loss.
i. What is seen in 157a and how has this changed by the time of the follow-up study (157b)?
ii. What is the likely histology?
iii. Are there any relevant aetiological factors?
iv. Could the management after the first endoscopy have been improved?

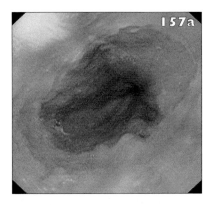

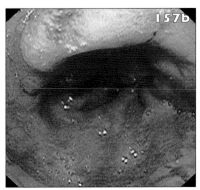

156 i. A leiomyoma. Leiomyomas, which arise from smooth muscle tissue, are the most common benign tumour of the stomach and are most frequently found incidentally at autopsy or surgery. They may ulcerate, as in this case, and hence are an uncommon cause of upper GI haemorrhage.
ii. These lesions are most often asymptomatic, especially the small tumours (<2 cm). The larger leiomyoma may present with GI bleeding as described above, or with recurrent abdominal pain. A further possible complication is malignant change. It may be difficult to distinguish the benign lesion from a malignant leiomyosarcoma. Treatment of symptomatic lesions consists of surgical resection and there have been no reported recurrences of benign lesions. The overall 5-year survival rate for leiomyosarcoma is 25–30%.

157 i. The first endoscopy (**157a**) revealed an area of Barrett's oesophagus, which is still apparent in the second image (**157b**), which shows the additional presence of a mass lesion and some contact bleeding.
ii. This is probably an adenocarcinoma (histology confirmed that it was).
iii. The presence of Barrett's oesophagus is an important aetiological factor in carcinoma of the distal oesophagus and one that is made more potent by smoking and heavy alcohol ingestion which are themselves also independent risk factors.
iv. It is probable that the malignancy was preceded by dysplasia and that endoscopic surveillance, with regular biopsies, might have permitted diagnosis at an earlier stage. At the very least, the area of Barrett's mucosa should have been biopsied on the first occasion, as dysplasia present at that time would have been a less controversial justification for surveillance than Barrett's alone. More intensive treatment with proton pump inhibitors may also have been influential in reducing the magnitude of inflammation, although it is yet to be proved whether this might have any effect in reducing the severity of dysplasia or the risk of carcinomatous transformation. The World Congress of Gastroenterology Working Party on Barrett's recommends endoscopy every 6 months if there is low-grade dysplasia or every 2 years if dysplasia is absent. Resection should always be seriously considered for those with high-grade dysplasia, as 33% of them otherwise develop carcinoma within 12 months.

158 A 64-year-old man complains of
progressive dysphagia for solids (158).
i. Describe the appearances shown in
158.
ii. Outline the pathogenesis.
iii. List the factors that may exacerbate
this condition.
iv. How might this patient be treated?

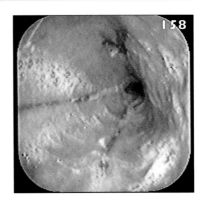

159 A 55-year-old man presents with
6 weeks of constant epigastric pain
radiating to the back; it is unrelieved
by NSAIDs and aspirin. He has lost
7 kg (15 lb) in weight. Physical
examination is unremarkable, with
the exception of epigastric fullness.
The upper endoscopy is completely
normal. A CT scan of the abdomen is
performed (159a).
i. Describe the abnormality present
on the CT scan.
ii. What additional diagnostic test
could be performed at the time of the
CT scan?
iii. PET is performed (159b). What is
the biochemical basis for this test,
and what is the implication of a
positive scan?
iv. The possibility of surgery is
discussed – what kind of surgery
would be required and what would
make this patient's disease unsuitable
for such an approach?

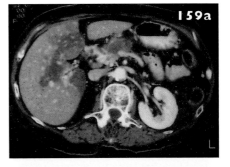

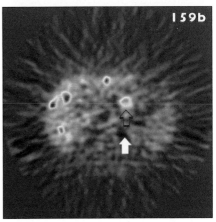

158 & 159: Answers

158 i. There is an oesophageal stricture with linear oesophagitis proximally (**158**).
ii. GORD results from:
- Failure of the reflux barrier mechanism at the oesophago-gastric junction, which is often disrupted by the presence of a hiatus hernia.
- Impaired oesophageal peristalsis; impaired salivary flow and delayed gastric emptying may aggravate a reflux tendency. A hiatus hernia also provides a reservoir of acid above the diaphragm.
- If acid reflux is severe and long-standing, a peptic stricture may eventually result.

iii. Exacerbating factors include:
Obesity, pregnancy, tight waistbands, coughing, smoking.

Food fats, chocolate, coffee, alcohol and peppermint reduce the resting LOS pressure, and increase the frequency of spontaneous sphincter relaxations.

Drugs – anticholinergics, nitrates, calcium antagonists, and theophylline derivatives relax the LOS. NSAIDs predispose to the development of strictures.

iv. Treatment should begin with lifestyle adjustments: weight loss, giving up smoking, raising the head of the bed, etc. Unfortunately, few patients comply.

Antacids are ineffective for healing, but are used primarily for symptom relief. Proton pump inhibitors are more effective than the H2 antagonists to effect symptom relief and healing, and frequently need to be taken long term to prevent relapse. Prokinetic agents (metoclopramide, domperidone, cisapride) variably increase the LOS pressure, stimulate oesophageal motility, and hasten gastric emptying.

The peptic stricture requires dilatation. A number of endoscopic techniques are available. Biopsy is performed to exclude malignancy. Subsequently, the patient remains on potent long-term anti-secretory therapy. Surgery is reserved for intractable symptoms despite optimal medical management.

159 i. A mass in the head of pancreas is seen; the likely diagnosis is adenocarcinoma of the pancreas. The 5-year survival rate is less than 5%.
ii. Fine needle aspiration biopsy may be performed under CT guidance. Rarely, the needle tract becomes seeded with tumour, so some clinicians prefer to proceed directly to laparotomy for otherwise potentially resectable lesions.
iii. PET depends on the uptake of ^{18}F-deoxyglucose (FDG) by the cellular glucose transport system. In normal cells, FDG is phosphorylated, then subsequently dephosphorylated. Malignant cells take up FDG avidly but are unable to dephosphorylate the FDG-6-phosphate. ^{18}F emits positrons which are detected by PET. The sensitivity and specificity appear to be high. False-positive scans are occasionally seen with pancreatitis. The arrow (**159b**) demonstrates a hot spot in the pancreatic head; the remaining spots are liver metastases.
iv. The only possible 'curative' surgery requires a Whipple procedure. All too often the tumour proves to be inoperable as the lesion may be more extensive than suggested by preoperative imaging. Invasion of adjacent vascular structures and metastases are clear contraindications. Palliative surgery for carcinoma of the head of pancreas usually requires a biliary diversion and a gastroenterostomy.

160 A 56-year-old engineer returned from
a 6-month trip to Africa complaining of
recurrent abdominal pain, diarrhoea and
weight loss.
i. What does this barium follow-through
examination show (160)?
ii. How would you confirm the diagnosis?
iii. What are the illness complications?
iv. What is the treatment?

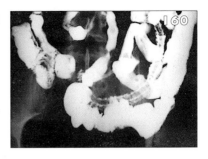

161 A 10-month-old baby has a 5-month history of diarrhoea. He was born
at term, breast fed since birth, and had a bowel frequency of more than five
times daily, with mustard–yellow stools. He was thriving and a weaning diet
was introduced at 4 months. Only after this did frothy, watery and explosive
stools develop. His family doctor advised a 24-hour period on oral
rehydration solution which stopped the diarrhoea, but when normal diet
was recommenced, so did the diarrhoea. The baby appeared well apart from
some perianal excoriation and mild abdominal distention. Stool pH was 5.0
and no reducing substances were present. During investigation the diarrhoea
stopped when he was on an intravenous infusion and kept fasted.
i. What is the most likely diagnosis?
ii. Which investigations would be most helpful?

162 A 28-year-old woman developed diarrhoea
and haematochezia 6 weeks after making, and
continuing to comply with, a New Year's
resolution to quit cigarette smoking. Flexible
sigmoidoscopy demonstrated superficial
ulcerations, loss of mucosal vascular pattern,
granularity, and a continuous inflammatory
process (162).
i. Are the onset of colitis and cessation of
cigarette smoking related?

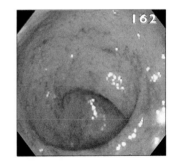

ii. Are cigarette smokers more likely to develop ulcerative colitis or Crohn's
disease?
iii. May smoking influence the course of established Crohn's disease?
iv. Should this patient start smoking again?
v. What is the mechanism for the influence of cigarette smoking on
inflammatory bowel disease?

160 –162: Answers

160 i. The follow-through (**160**) shows a filling defect in the mid-ileum. It has the appearances of *Ascaris lumbricoides*.
ii. The diagnosis was confirmed by the identification of ova in a fresh, warm stool sample.
iii. Although uncomplicated in this patient, *Ascaris* infections may present with intestinal obstruction. Worms can cause biliary colic and obstruction. After ingestion, the fertilized eggs hatch in the duodenum and the larvae penetrate the intestinal wall, migrate to the lungs, penetrate through the alveolar wall and ascend the trachea and are subsequently swallowed to complete their development into mature females in the intestine. Larvae migrating in the lungs may cause both pulmonary hypersensitivity and pulmonary infiltrates with an eosinophilia (Loeffler's syndrome).
iv. This patient was successfully treated with mebendazole, though pyrantel pamoate or piperazine citrate are also appropriate.

161 i. He has an osmotic non-secretory diarrhoea as supported by the curtailment of the diarrhoea whenever fasted. There is no evidence of impaired absorption of monosaccharides, and the normal growth and generally good development exclude many of the metabolic disorders. The most likely diagnosis is therefore congenital sucrose–isomaltase deficiency.
ii. Diagnosis is confirmed by stool chromatography, sucrose tolerance test and disaccharidase assay of a small-bowel biopsy.

This is an autosomal recessive condition with absent intestinal sucrase and reduced isomaltase; it is common only in Greenland. It usually presents as soon as sucrose is introduced into the infant's diet, but may not be a problem until later childhood. Lifelong avoidance of sucrose is required to avoid symptoms, but the prognosis is otherwise good.

162 i. Consistent epidemiological studies have linked cigarette smoking to the development of inflammatory bowel disease. Quitters are more likely than non-smokers to develop ulcerative colitis. This woman developed ulcerative colitis soon after stopping to smoke, which is a commonly encountered scenario.
ii. Cigarette smokers are more likely to develop Crohn's disease and appear to be protected from developing ulcerative colitis.
iii. Smokers with Crohn's disease are predisposed to a more severe course than non-smokers with Crohn's disease, and have a greater relapse rate after surgery.
iv. The adverse effects of cigarette smoking on bodily functions and cancer risk are legion. However, trials of nicotine patches to treat patients with ulcerative colitis have confirmed short-term benefits in those who can tolerate the side effects. Long-term, or maintenance therapy beyond 8 weeks, has not been shown to be helpful and can lead to nicotine addiction.
v. The mechanism remains unknown but may be due to an effect on mucus integrity and/or inflammatory mediators.

163 A 71-year-old man presents with intermittent food-related epigastric discomfort. He has vomited on occasion but has not lost any weight. He denies any prior illnesses. He takes the occasional aspirin. His symptoms continue despite a 6-week course of H2-receptor antagonists. The patient's physician reports that a barium meal (upper GI series) demonstrates a filling defect in the gastric antrum, but the films are not available at the time of the consultation. Physical examination is normal but the stools are slightly positive for the presence of occult blood. The complete blood count is normal. An upper endoscopy demonstrates a pedunculated 2 cm polyp with a smooth but lobulated surface close to the pylorus (163a).

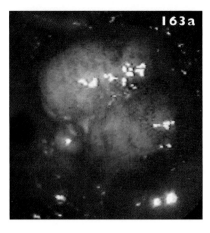

i. Are the patient's symptoms attributable to the endoscopic findings?
ii. Speculate on the likelihood of gastric cancer being present.
iii. How should the endoscopist proceed?
iv. Discuss the differential diagnosis of benign gastric polypoid lesions and their risk for malignancy.
v. Is follow-up necessary?

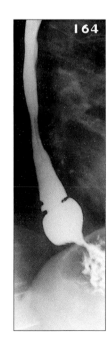

164 This barium swallow examination (164) was performed in a reasonably healthy 45-year-old man.
i. What is the abnormality?
ii. What is the differential diagnosis?
iii. What were his most likely symptoms?
iv. What, if any, useful treatment is available?

163 & 164: Answers

163 i. It is likely that he has experienced intermittent pyloric obstruction.
ii. Endoscopically gastric adenocarcinoma usually presents as a mass or ulcerated lesion. A pedunculated polyp with a smooth surface is a less likely presentation.
iii. Pedunculated lesions are generally easily removed. If standard sampling of a suspicious lesion demonstrates malignancy, a surgical approach is justified. Injection of saline into the base of more broad-based lesions may enhance the safety of endoscopic removal. Endoscopic ultrasound may facilitate the evaluation.

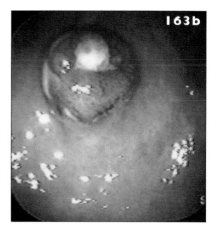
163b

iv. Adenomatous polyps are predominantly solitary and found in the antrum. Malignant potential increases as the size of the polyp increases. Hyperplastic polyps are more commonly <1 cm in diameter and randomly situated. Up to 2% undergo malignant degeneration. Gastric carcinoids are found, mainly proximally, in 4% of patients with pernicious anaemia. Inflammatory polyps have also been associated with adenocarcinoma. All polyps may ulcerate (163b) and bleed, and, if strategically situated, lead to obstructive symptoms.
v. The cost-effectiveness of follow-up of completely removed benign gastric polyps is unknown.

164 i. There is a narrowing in the distal oesophagus
ii. This is probably the result of a Schatski ring, but oesophageal webs can also have this radiological appearance. Neoplastic strictures are usually less regular, and there are no suggestions of the associated chronic reflux oesophagitis and stenosis to be expected with a benign 'peptic' stricture. Webs may occur at any site in the oesophagus and usually contain mucosa and submucosa, but no muscle. Those of the Plummer–Vinson syndrome, associated with iron-deficiency anaemia and an increased risk of hypopharyngeal carcinoma, occur at the junction of the upper and middle thirds of the oesophagus. Oesophageal rings are generally thicker structures which may contain some muscle.
iii. Webs and rings are usually asymptomatic, but can be responsible for dysphagia, especially if the residual lumen is <12 mm. The dysphagia is usually intermittent, but may be dramatic if a food bolus becomes impacted.
iv. Diagnostic endoscopy is very often therapeutic, as the passage of a standard-calibre endoscope through the area of narrowing is almost always very easy and may be sufficient to cause permanent disruption of the ring or web. Formal balloon or bougie dilatation is rarely required.

165 A 60-year-old alcoholic cirrhotic complains of difficulty seeing at night, especially when driving and facing oncoming headlights. An evaluation by his local ophthalmologist included a dark adaptation study (**165**).
i. Based on the history and the dark adaptation study, what is the patient's problem?
ii. What nutritional deficiency is likely to be causing this problem?
iii. Why might this patient have this nutritional inadequacy?
iv. How would you treat him?
v. What are the potential complications of therapy in this patient?

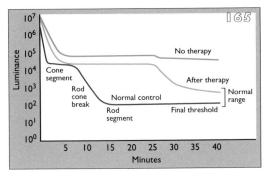

166 A 63-year-old male presents to the emergency room with a history of left lower quadrant pain that came on suddenly early that morning. The patient had experienced similar attacks in the past that were not as severe and were treated by his family doctor with antibiotics and low-fibre diet. He also has had several loose bowel movements without seeing any blood. Two days earlier he had eaten peanuts at a baseball game. He has been in good health and had a colonoscopy 3 years earlier for faecal occult positive stool. Apart from the findings demonstrated in **166a**, no other abnormalities were detected then. Examination revealed a patient in considerable distress. His temperature was 39°C, blood pressure 152/90 mmHg, pulse 110/min. Bowel sounds were decreased in frequency and high-pitched. A questionable fullness was felt in the left lower quadrant that produced localized rebound tenderness. Laboratory data were significant for a leukocyte count of 13.4×10^9/l (13 400/mm^3) with 16% bands and 62% polymorphonuclear leukocytes.
i. Describe the endoscopic abnormality shown (**166a**).
ii. What is the most likely diagnosis at this visit?
iii. How may the diagnosis best be confirmed?
iv. What treatment is appropriate at this time?
v. Comment on possible complications of this disorder.

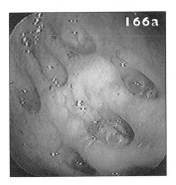

165 & 166: Answers

165 i. The patient has night blindness.
ii. Vitamin A deficiency. Vitamin A is necessary for the generation of visual purple (rhodopsin), which is required for normal rod function and night vision. Vitamin A combines with specific proteins called opsins to form the photosensitive visual pigments of rods and cones. With vitamin A deficiency, rhodopsin levels decline; the rod threshold increases and night blindness occurs.
iii. Poor dietary intake, malabsorption, impaired hepatic storage (depletion may take up to 2 years), and decreased synthesis and release of retinol-binding protein.
iv. With low-dose vitamin A supplementation (about 5000–10 000 units vitamin A, or 1500–3000 g/day) for approximately 1 month. Improvement in dark adaptation may then be re-assessed. If improved, the patient should consume a well-balanced diet with the possible addition of a multi-vitamin containing the RDA of vitamin A (**165**).
v. Vitamin A toxicity produces liver damage, headache, nausea and vomiting, diplopia, alopecia and dry mucous membranes. Patients with underlying liver disease and low retinol-binding protein levels, as well as those with renal impairment, may be more susceptible to vitamin A toxicity.

166 i. Multiple diverticula.
ii. The patient has intra-abdominal sepsis, with diverticulitis being the most likely cause.
iii. CT scanning is replacing barium enema as the study of choice because of the concern that barium installation may lead to a free perforation. Furthermore, the scan may readily diagnose abscess formation. Endoscopic procedures are avoided during acute diverticulitis.
iv. Bed rest, bowel rest, intravenous fluids, and antibiotics that cover *Bacteroides fragilis* and *Escherichia coli*. Between 70% and 85% of patients recover and the remainder require surgery. Phlegmonous peridiverticulitis resolves with prolonged antimicrobial therapy. Abscess formation (**166b** depicts air in a diverticula abscess) is an indication for percutaneous drainage and/or surgery. Surgery for perforation or

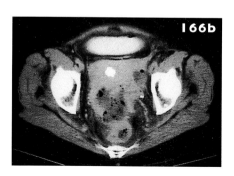
166b

sepsis invariably requires a temporary diversion procedure. Consideration of elective resection of the involved area should be given for recurrent diverticulitis or other chronic symptoms.
v. Diverticulitis; inflammatory stricture and fistulization with the genitourinary tract and small bowel may also occur. Other complications include abscess, peritonitis and portal pyaemia. Right-sided diverticulitis may mimic appendicitis.

167 A 50-year-old man experienced mid-abdominal pain and a tendency to loose stools. He noted periodic flushing accompanied by lightheadedness. Physical examination is notable for an enlarged nodular liver. The ALP is 315 u/l (normal <110 u/l). A barium study reveals an irregular mass in the distal ileum. An abdominal CT scan demonstrates hepatomegaly with multiple hypodense lesions (**167**).

The AFP is not elevated.

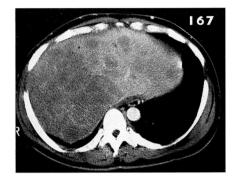

i. What does the CT scan suggest?
ii. Which tumour is likely?
iii. How does the presence of this tumour explain the patient's symptoms and physical findings?
iv. Discuss the biochemistry of this disorder.
v. Which treatment options should be considered?

168 A 58-year-old woman presents with a history of left-sided abdominal discomfort, bloating and a change in bowel habit, but with no rectal bleeding or weight loss. She was on treatment for her asthma. Sigmoidoscopy (**168a**) and plain abdominal radiograph (**168b**) are shown.

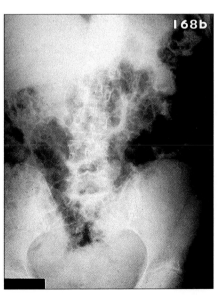

i. What diagnosis is suggested?
ii. Name some of the associations of this condition.
iii. Outline its treatment.

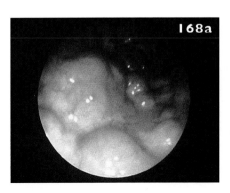

167 & 168: Answers

167 i. Metastatic disease. Hepatocellular carcinoma is unlikely as the AFP is normal.
ii. Small-bowel carcinoid metastatic to the liver.
iii. The carcinoid syndrome occurs when liver dysfunction due to metastatic disease fails to inactivate tumour-derived proteins. The most common symptom experienced is flushing. Moderate diarrhoea may occur. Right-sided endomyocardial fibrosis of the tricuspid and pulmonary valves and bronchoconstriction present late in the course of the disease. Abdominal symptoms may be due to luminal narrowing by the tumour or the cicatrizing effect of proteins elaborated by the tumour. An obliterative arteritis may result in local ischaemia.
iv. Carcinoid tumours synthesize serotonin, which is metabolized to 5-HIAA. 5-HIAA accesses the systemic circulation if it bypasses hepatic inactivation. High 5-HIAA levels are present in patients with the carcinoid syndrome. Prostaglandins and bradykinin have vasodilating properties and probably cause the flushing.
v. Surgery should be considered for resectable localized disease, and for intestinal obstruction. Chemotherapy may be useful in reducing tumour bulk. Octreotide controls many of the clinical manifestations.

168 i. Pneumatosis coli.
ii. Necrotizing enterocolitis, COAD, pyloric stenosis, systemic sclerosis, ischaemic bowel, immunosuppressive agents, vasculitis, colitis.
   It is an uncommon condition in which gas-filled cysts are found in the submucosa and subserosa of the bowel. It is important to differentiate the benign asymptomatic form – which usually settles with oxygen – from a potentially life-threatening symptomatic form associated with perforation, infection, and ischaemia which requires immediate surgery.
   The cysts can mimic polyps on sigmoidoscopy.
   168b reveals air in the bowel wall. **168a** demonstrates cysts with a bluish tinge. When punctured, they deflate with a popping sound.

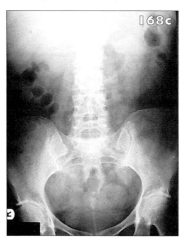

iii. Management depends on the underlying cause and the patient's symptoms. It is generally asymptomatic and runs a benign course. If symptomatic, various treatment options exist:
* High-concentration oxygen via face mask.
* Hyperbaric oxygen has also been advocated.
* The efficacy of antibiotics is not established.
* A low-residue diet may limit fermentation and minimize gas production.
* Surgery – this is very rarely warranted unless features suggest an imminent catastrophe, e.g. portal venous gas on the plain abdominal radiograph, or bowel infarction apparent clinically. The condition may relapse after apparently successful medical therapy (**168c**).

169 A 50-year-old man presents for a
general medical evaluation. A flexible
sigmoidoscopy is performed for screening
purposes. At 35 cm from the anal verge, a
2 cm diameter lesion (169) is encountered.
i. What is the probable nature of the lesion
encountered?
ii. Should a biopsy be performed?
iii. Which treatment is most appropriate?
iv. Describe further management strategies.
v. Comment on the association of colon
adenomas with other non-syndromic
disorders.

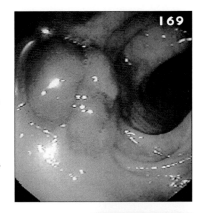

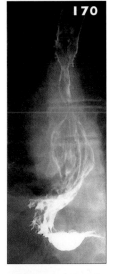

170 An elderly woman presented with a gradually
worsening history of heartburn and regurgitation, weight
loss of 2 kg (4.5 lb) and a troublesome cough.
i. What does the barium swallow (170) demonstrate?
ii. What are the likely causes?
iii. How should this patient be managed?

171 A patient, who is asymptomatic, attended
for a screening endoscopy. 171 shows the
colonoscopic appearance of her colon.
i. What is the clinical diagnosis that is most
likely?
ii. What is the treatment of choice for this
condition?
iii. What is the likely outcome for patients
who decline treatment?
iv. Give two other clinical conditions that can
occur in this disease.
v. Describe the genetic abnormality.

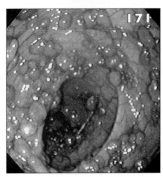

169 i. Adenomatous polyp with little evidence of pedunculation.
ii. It is cost-effective to biopsy small lesions and to proceed directly to colonoscopic removal of larger ones. While a significant proportion of diminutive lesions constitute hyperplastic polyps, the majority of large lesions are adenomatous.
iii. The colon is examined for synchronous lesions, and all polyps removed. Sigmoid colectomy is indicated only if the polyp proves to be malignant with invasive features, or if the polyp is too sessile with a broad base as here.
iv. Surveillance colonoscopy at 3 years to search for metachronous lesions. Thereafter, given normal findings, surveillance intervals may be extended. A reduced-fat, fibre-enhanced diet may be useful.
v. Acromegaly is associated with an increased prevalence of colonic adenomas, and ureterosigmoidostomy sites are at increased risk for colorectal neoplasia. Colon tumours may predispose to *Streptococcus bovis* bacteraemia.

170 i. A smooth oesophageal narrowing in the lower third, above a hiatus hernia. There is food residue and pseudo-diverticula.
ii. Benign peptic stricture associated with long-standing reflux disease. However, neoplasia cannot be absolutely excluded. A pre-existing Barrett's oesophagus could be present.
iii. Malignancy is best excluded by endoscopy, with cytology and biopsies. With a benign disorder, dilatation with bougies or balloons is then appropriate. Long-term acid suppression with a proton pump inhibitor is required as well as lifestyle changes, e.g. stopping smoking, weight reduction, and raising the head of the bed. Surgery is considered for medically intractable symptoms or malignancy.

171 i. Familial adenomatous polyposis (FAP), characterized by the presence of hundreds of adenomatous polyps throughout the colon. There is a more than 90% probability of a positive sigmoidoscopy by the age of 25 years if the person being screened has inherited (autosomal dominant) the abnormal gene. Sporadic cases can occur as new mutations.
ii. Surgery is the only reasonable option for patients with FAP, once colonic polyps have been identified – colectomy with ileorectal anastomosis, or panproctocolectomy and ileoanal anastomosis. The former procedure has a continuing risk of developing rectal carcinoma.
iii. Without a colectomy, all patients eventually develop colorectal cancer at an average age of 40–45 years.
iv. Extra-colonic features are now recognized to be common in FAP patients and include hyperplastic polyps in the stomach, duodenal and periampullary adenomas and carcinoma, and congenital hypertrophy of the retinal pigment epithelium (CHRPE). Some manifestations are more evident in Gardner's syndrome, including osteomas, desmoid tumours, dental abnormalities, epidermoid and sebaceous cysts, lipomas and fibromas, plus non-colonic neoplasms, in particular thyroid carcinoma.
v. The gene responsible is the *APC* gene. The mutation is present on the long arm of chromosome 5 (5q21) and can vary from family to family, although it always runs true within the same family.

172 A segment of intestine (172) was
resected from an 18-year-old woman
with acute onset of right lower quadrant
pain, fever, nausea, and vomiting believed
to indicate acute appendicitis.
i. What is the pathological lesion (172)?
ii. What is the likely diagnosis?
iii. Which other disorders may result in
similar pathological appearances?
iv. Is surgery curative?
v. Is therapy useful to maintain a surgically induced remission?

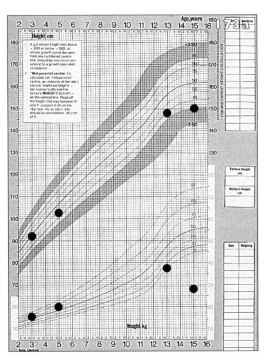

173 A 15-year-old girl was admitted
with a 4-year history of non-bilious
vomiting, recurrent abdominal pain
and extreme weight loss (173a is her
growth chart). She had been treated
for duodenal ulceration seen
endoscopically about 2 years before,
with a regime based on bismuth and
antibiotics. The social circumstances
were poor – the girl shared a three-
roomed local authority apartment
with her parents and 11 siblings. On
examination she was emaciated, pale,
with poor dental hygiene, and
prepubertal. Abdominal examination
revealed tenderness in the epigastrium
and a succussion splash. Further
endoscopy revealed an oedematous
pylorus and duodenal ulcer; an antral
biopsy was obtained (173b).
i. What is the differential diagnosis?
ii. In what way, if any, is the antral

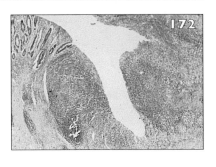

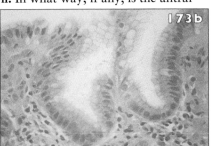

biopsy helpful?
iii. Endoscopy showed a significant
degree of pyloric oedema; it was
possible to pass the instrument into
the duodenum nevertheless and only a
single duodenal ulcer was identified.
What therapeutic interventions
might now be suggested?

163

172 & 173: Answers

172 i. Terminal ileum demonstrating a non-caseating granuloma next to a deep fissure.
ii. Granulomata are found in 20–60% of patients with Crohn's disease. Many young patients with Crohn's disease first present with acute abdominal pain, frequently in the right lower quadrant, as well as fever, weight loss, and a palpable mass.
iii. Sarcoidosis, tuberculosis, histoplasmosis, fungal infections, schistosomiasis and actinomycosis may present with intestinal granulomata, but have different clinical presentations.
iv. Unfortunately, relapses following surgery are very frequent.
v. Remissions may last for several years, although disease tends to recur at the site of surgical anastomosis. High-dose mesalamine (mesalazine) appears beneficial for maintaining remission. In aggressive disease with early (<3 months) post-surgical recurrences, immunosuppressive drugs (azathioprine or 6-mercaptopurine) may be helpful in maintaining remission.

173 i. The differential diagnosis includes gastric outlet obstruction due to a recurrent duodenal ulcer and Zollinger–Ellison syndrome. Abdominal lymphoma is also a possibility. In the presence of severe social deprivation, failure to thrive may also be seen – and be responsible for non-specific pains and failure of growth and sexual maturation.
ii. The antral biopsy (**173b**) shows a chronic inflammatory infiltrate with *H. pylori*.
iii. Given the importance of now ensuring eradication of *H. pylori*, a urea breath test 6 weeks after completing a course that included a proton pump inhibitor and two antibiotics (e.g. amoxycillin, clarithromycin and omeprazole) should be performed. Anti-secretory therapy should be continued for another month. Pyloric dilatation could be considered if obstructive symptoms persist. Serum gastrin should be measured.

174 A 78-year-old man hospitalized with dysphagia due to a cerebrovascular accident had acute onset of upper abdominal pain, vomiting and slight diarrhoea. He was pyrexial (38°C) but not jaundiced. There was no lymphadenopathy. On abdominal examination, he was tender in the right upper quadrant with some guarding. A plain abdominal film was taken (174).
i. What abnormality is seen in 174?
ii. What is this appearance due to?
iii. What other investigations might you wish to carry out?

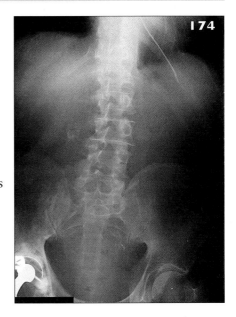

175 A 45-year-old man presents with postprandial epigastric pain, diarrhoea and ankle swelling. The blood count, liver enzymes and urinalysis are normal. The serum albumin is 23 g/l (normal, 35–58 g/l). Endoscopy reveals hypertrophic gastric folds (175a), which are biopsied (175b). The gastric pH is 4.0. His fasting serum gastrin level is 234 pg/ml (normal, <100 pg/ml).
i. What conditions cause epigastric pain, hypertrophic folds and elevated serum gastrin levels?
ii. What condition does he have and how can the diagnosis be confirmed?
iii. Why does he have oedema of the ankles?
iv. Discuss treatment.

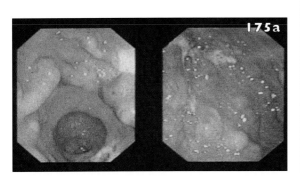
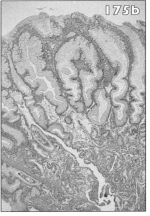

174 i. In the right upper quadrant, multiple faceted radio-opaque lesions can be seen along with some calcification of the gallbladder (and a nasogastric tube).
ii. The radio-opaque nature of gallstones is due to their calcium content. About 10% are radio-opaque. Only 10% of cholesterol stones are radio-opaque, while up to 60% of black pigment stones can be seen on plain abdominal radiographs.
iii. It is probable that the symptoms are of biliary origin. Scintigraphic biliary excretion scanning may help to clarify this, as may ultrasound scanning which also determines whether there is biliary obstruction – and therefore a justification for early ERCP and sphincterotomy. A chest radiography excludes respiratory infection, aspiration being possible given the neurology. Other causes of abdominal pain such as peptic ulcer, acute pancreatitis and mesenteric ischaemia are also considered.

175 i. The differential diagnosis of gastric rugal hyperrugosity includes proliferation of the parietal cell mass (seen in Zollinger–Ellison syndrome, hypertrophic hypersecretory gastropathy and *H. pylori* gastritis), diffuse infiltrative processes (such as occurs in gastric carcinoma, lymphoma, eosinophilic gastritis and amyloidosis) and Ménétrier's disease. Although Zollinger–Ellison syndrome is associated with elevations of fasting serum gastrin and gastric acid hypersecretion, the gastric pH in this case is >3.0. Hypertrophic hypersecretory gastropathy has elevated gastric acid secretion but an appropriately normal serum gastrin. Diffuse infiltrative processes may be associated with appropriately elevated serum gastrin levels due to loss of parietal cells, but such infiltration should be apparent on biopsy.
ii. In Ménétrier's disease, the gastric folds are large due to replacement of the parietal (and chief) cells by an expanded gastric foveolar mass. This may be confirmed by a deep biopsy (175b). Gastric acid secretion may therefore be reduced and an appropriate hypergastrinaemia occurs. This disorder is of unknown aetiology and generally occurs in men. A similar (albeit self-limiting) syndrome due to cytomegalovirus gastritis has been described in children.
iii. Ménétrier's disease is typically associated with hypoalbuminaemia due to a protein-losing gastropathy. Peripheral oedema is common. Enteric loss of protein may be confirmed by testing stool for alpha-1-antitrypsin. Protein-losing enteropathy from infiltrative processes in the small bowel (such as lymphoma, lymphangiectasia, or amyloidosis) are other possible causes for the hypoalbuminaemia and pedal oedema in this patient, but these conditions are not associated with hypergastrinaemia and foveolar hyperplasia on endoscopic biopsy. Non-enteric causes of hypoalbuminaemia and oedema include poor protein intake, chronic liver disease, and proteinuria.
iv. Some patients with subclinical disease may do well with supportive therapy. Antisecretory agents have no established role. Gastric resection may ultimately be required to control the protein loss. Gastric adenocarcinoma has been reported to be a complication.

176 A 56-year-old man presents with
abdominal pain and weight loss. He is found
to have a mass palpable in the epigastrium,
and a pigmented skin thickening involving
both axillae (176).
i. What is this skin lesion?
ii. Comment on associated disorders.
iii. Is biopsy indicated?
iv. Comment on the temporal relationships
of this lesion to malignant disease.

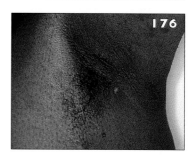

v. Discuss other cutaneous signs of gastrointestinal malignancy.

177 A 45-year-old man with a history of
peptic ulcer disease presents to his doctor
for complaints of progressive fatigue and
mild dyspnoea on exertion. The stool is
brown and the faecal occult blood is
positive. A routine blood count reveals that
haemoglobin is 8.0 g/dl and haematocrit is
24%. Erythrocytes are microcytic and there
is no evidence of haemolysis on peripheral
blood smear. Colonoscopy and
oesophagogastroduodenoscopy are both
normal. A small-bowel follow-through
(177a) is also normal.
i. What diagnoses are considered in this
case?
ii. What further work-up is considered?
iii. Comment on the abnormality seen in
177b.
iv. What is the pathogenesis and natural
history of this lesion?
v. What confirmatory testing and treatment
may be appropriate?

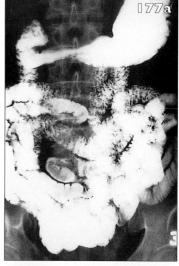

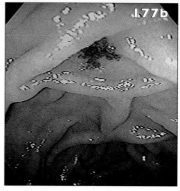

176 & 177: Answers

176 i. Acanthosis nigricans.
ii. It is most commonly seen in obese individuals, with insulin resistance, but may be familial. The possible presence of an intra-abdominal or intrapelvic malignancy, particularly gastric adenocarcinoma, should be entertained.
iii. Biopsy of the lesion is not helpful.
iv. It may precede the appearance of a malignancy by many years. A tumour search includes upper and lower endoscopic evaluation, and CT scanning of the abdomen and pelvis. The skin lesion may remit after the tumour has been removed. Its appearance in a patient known to have an adenocarcinoma often heralds recurrent or metastatic disease.
v. Tumours may involve the skin indirectly via the release of chemical mediators as in the carcinoid (flushing) and glucagonoma (necrolytic migratory erythema) syndromes. Other manifestations of malignancy include keratoderma (tylosis), and hypertrichosis lanuginosa acquisita. Secondary nutritional deficiencies may also produce skin lesions. Colonic polyposis syndromes are also associated with cutaneous lesions, including melanotic macules (Peutz–Jeghers syndrome), epidermoid cysts (Gardner's syndrome), hyperpigmentation, alopecia and onychodystrophy (Cronkhite–Canada syndrome), papules, café au lait macules (Cowden's disease) and sebaceous neoplasms, and keratoacanthomas (Muir–Torre syndrome).

177 i. This patient has gastrointestinal bleeding of obscure origin. Endoscopy may occasionally overlook vascular ectasias or the rare Dieulafoy's lesion which generally presents with intermittent, usually massive, upper GI bleeding resulting from an ectatic vessel which has eroded through the mucosa of the gastric fundus. A number of small-bowel lesions (including small-bowel vascular ectasias, Meckel's diverticulum, and small neoplasms) may be difficult to detect.
ii. Bleeding scans (scintigraphy) are usually unhelpful unless bleeding is clinically active. Direct inspection of the small bowel may be achieved by enteroscopy. Angiography may detect an abnormal vasculature, even if no active haemorrhage is occurring.
iii. Small-bowel vascular ectasia.
iv. Vascular ectasias (angiodysplasias) are acquired lesions that probably result from chronic low-grade obstruction of submucosal veins. Pathology reveals dilated, distorted, thin-walled vessels lined by epithelium alone or by epithelium with a small amount of smooth muscle. Vascular ectasias are found most often in the colon. They frequently lie close to the luminal surface and may be associated with either massive or occult GI bleeding.
v. Angiography may reveal a vascular tuft during the intra-arterial phase of the study, as well as early venous filling. The vein may be dilated and may be slow to empty. Angiography, if performed during a bleeding episode, may also demonstrate extravasation of contrast into the bowel. Treatment of symptomatic vascular ectasias consists of ablation by means of cautery, or laser therapy for endoscopically accessible lesions. Surgery may be required for endoscopic failures, particularly for localized lesions. Long-term oral hormone therapy may decrease transfusional requirements.

178 A 65-year-old alcoholic smoker presents with a 10 kg weight loss over the previous 2 months because of progressive dysphagia, first for solids and now both for solids and liquids. He summoned an ambulance because he had become too dizzy and weak on standing to walk. Examination demonstrated a wasted, unkempt and dehydrated elderly man. Attempts to swallow liquid result in regurgitation within minutes. An endoscopy was performed but the instrument could not be advanced beyond a lesion in the distal oesophagus (178a).
i. Describe the endoscopic appearances in 178a.
ii. What additional diagnostic testing may help?
iii. Comment on the risk factors for this lesion.
iv. Discuss nutritional management.
v. Discuss management of the lesion.

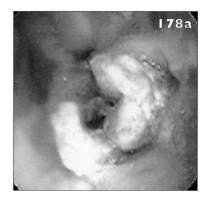

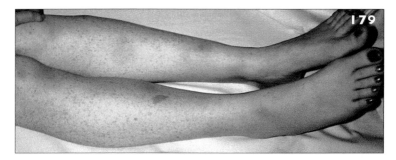

179 A 26-year-old female (179) had been diagnosed with Crohn's disease 4 years earlier. Over the previous 2 years she had required intermittent then continuous therapy with steroids. She had been started on azathioprine 3 weeks before and her steroids had been reduced from 15 mg to 5 mg per day. Her stool frequency had increased from three soft stools per day to four to six. She also reported arthralgia and a recent sore throat.
i. What is the skin lesion in 179?
ii. In what way might it be related to her therapy?
iii. What other investigations should be carried out?
iv. How should she be treated?

178 i. Endoscopy demonstrates an obstructing mass, probably a squamous carcinoma. Adenocarcinoma of the oesophagus arises from Barrett's epithelium, or proximal spread of a gastric lesion.

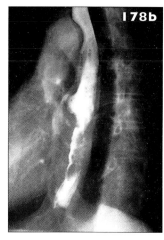

ii. The lesion is biopsied and brushings taken for cytology. A barium swallow helps determine the length of the stricture (178b), and rules out a gastric origin. CT scanning and endoscopic ultrasound help staging.
iii. Alcohol, tobacco abuse, caustic and radiation injury, incompletely treated achalasia, nasopharangeal tumours and tylosis.
iv. An optimal nutritional state may be difficult to attain. Endoscopic dilatation, tumour ablation with laser or electrocautery may allow placement of a gastrostomy device or oesophageal prosthesis (178c). Photodynamic therapy is being evaluated.

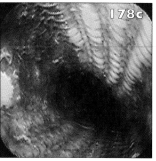

v. Metastatic disease is found at diagnosis in 85% of cases. Treatment options include a combination of surgery, radiotherapy and chemotherapy. The optimal treatment regimen has not been determined. Surgery provides the only modality for cure of localized lesions. The 5-year survival rate is 6%.

179 i. 179 shows erythema nodosum. There are numerous causes, although the co-existence of Crohn's disease makes this the likeliest, particularly as it is associated with an increase in Crohn's disease activity.
ii. The steroids may have been reduced too quickly after the commencement of azathioprine, which takes 8–12 weeks to reach its maximal effect. The presence of a sore throat while taking azathioprine means an FBC is essential to check for bone marrow suppression. This should be done weekly for the first 2 weeks, 2-weekly for a month after starting and then every 4–6 weeks for as long as the drug is continued.
iii. Although less likely, the combination of a recent sore throat, arthralgia and erythema nodosum should always stimulate exclusion of rheumatic fever; thus, antistreptolysin titres and an ECG should also be requested in this patient.
iv. The steroid dose should be increased until the azathioprine takes effect. An alternative, or additional therapy would be a course of metronidazole 400 mg which is continued for 1–2 months.

180 A 60-year-old woman presented with urinary frequency, dysuria and nocturia. She admitted to weight loss of about 3 kg (7 lb) over the preceding 2 months. Her friends had commented that they thought she looked 'a little yellow'.
i. What examination (**180**) has been performed?
ii. What abnormality does it show?
iii. What other features should be sought in the history and on examination?

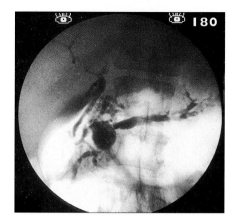

181 A 64-year-old man presents with weight loss, early satiety, postprandial bloating, nausea and intermittent vomiting which has become progressively severe over recent weeks. He noticed partially digested food, consumed the previous day, in the vomitus. He recalls some indigestion many years previously but denies any known previous peptic disease or non-steroidal anti-inflammatory drug use. Examination reveals a thin man without any lymphadenopathy, and a tenderness to deep palpation in the epigastrium. There is a fullness but no mass in this area. A succussion splash is present. The blood count is normal but there is hypokalaemia and a reduced serum albumin. An upper endoscopy reveals partially digested food in the stomach. The instrument is unable to negotiate the pylorus, which appears narrowed and irregular (**181a**). The stomach is otherwise normal.
i. What is the mechanical problem and its probable aetiology?
ii. What is the significance of the hypokalaemia and hypoalbuminaemia?
iii. What is the role of acid suppressive therapy (either H2-receptor or proton pump blockers) at this stage?
iv. Comment on additional investigations that may be useful in this case.
v. Comment on possible treatment strategies.

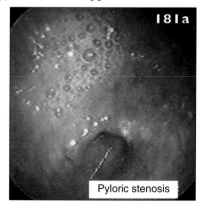

Pyloric stenosis

171

180 i. The examination is an ERCP.
ii. It shows an irregular dilated pancreatic duct with few side branches and a cyst in the head of the gland. The biliary tree is normal. These are the appearances of chronic pancreatitis. A first presentation with diabetes mellitus is not unusual. Patients may also present with obstructive jaundice if an inflammatory enlargement of the pancreatic head or pseudocyst causes obstruction of the common bile duct. Although the ERCP shows no evidence of this in the present case, it is possible that the questioned jaundice was from this cause and that the degree of inflammation had diminished by the time of the examination.
iii. The single most important feature of the history is alcohol consumption. Alcohol excess accounts for the huge majority of cases of chronic pancreatitis in most centres. Other causes, such as pancreas divisum, hereditary pancreatitis, and disorder of the sphincter of Oddi, may be suggested by the history. The many causes of acute pancreatitis rarely if ever lead on to chronic disease. Examination may be helpful by revealing cutaneous or other signs of liver disease, by the presence of a steatorrhoeic stool, and less often by the presence of a palpable mass related to the pancreas.

181 i. Gastric outlet obstruction due to pyloric stenosis. Peptic ulcer disease involving the pylorus or duodenum, either active immediately downstream of the narrowed area, or inactive with cicatrization, is the most probable aetiology. A gastric cancer causing obstruction without a mass lesion being visible is unusual.
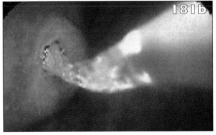
ii. They result from loss of acid due to vomiting. Hypoalbuminaemia suggests malnutrition.
iii. A mechanical problem exists, but is unlikely to benefit from acid suppression alone.
iv. The stenotic area is biopsied and a test for *H. pylori* performed. A barium examination to determine the anatomy downstream of the narrowing seldom provides strategic information. A CT scan is performed if extrinsic compression or tumour is suspected. Hypergastrinaemia is common in gastric outlet obstruction and may not imply the presence of a gastrinoma.
v. An attempt to dilate the pylorus endoscopically (**181b**) may succeed. If unsuccessful, a nasogastric tube is placed to decompress the stomach to improve mural tone. Intravenous fluids and nutrition must be provided if nasoenteral tube placement cannot be accomplished. Intravenous H2-receptor antagonists may be administered. A repeat attempt at endoscopic dilatation may be attempted later, followed by surgery if unsuccessful. Long-term results of endoscopic treatment of pyloric stenosis are disappointing.

182 Answer TRUE or FALSE to each of the following statements regarding intestinal absorption.

i. Every day around 9 l of endogenously produced fluid is presented to the luminal absorptive surface.

ii. Individual anatomic properties each increase the surface area for absorption by up to a factor of 20.

iii. Unlike jejunal absorption of sodium chloride, which occurs by a carrier-mediated mechanism, ileal absorption of sodium chloride occurs by passive diffusion.

iv. Sodium absorption is accelerated by altered carrier affinity for sodium and hydrogen by non-electrolyte molecules.

v. Sodium chloride absorption by the colon is stimulated by aldosterone.

183 A 38-year-old man with insulin-dependent diabetes since the age of 10 years has episodic watery diarrhoea for 18 months, which wakes him at night. He passes a watery, brown stool up to 10 times a day. He denies pain, vomiting or weight loss. His diabetes is well controlled on insulin and his only chronic complication is mild diabetic eye disease. He is on no additional regular medication. Examination reveals mild peripheral oedema and diminished pin-prick sensation in both feet. The abdomen is neither tender nor distended. Rectal examination is normal; BUN 6.8 mmol/l (19 mg/dl); creatinine 88 μmol/l (1.2 mg/dl); Na 136 mmol/l; K 3.5 mmol/l; bilirubin 12 μmol/l (0.7 mg/dl); albumin 30 g/l; SGPT 24 u/l; ALP 128 u/l (normal 75–150 u/l). Haemoglobin is 11.9 g/dl, MCV 98 fl, serum B_{12} 84 pmol/l (normal 150–400 pmol/l). However, despite weekly injections of 1000 μg vitamin B_{12} for 3 months, the haematological indices remain unaltered. Three-day faecal fat = 14 g (normal). Barium follow-through and abdominal CT scan are normal. In **183**, Series 1 shows a glucose hydrogen breath test after ingestion of 50 g glucose. Series 2 shows the result 2 weeks after a therapeutic intervention which rendered the patient symptom-free.

i. What is the diagnosis and therapeutic intervention utilized?

ii. List the possible causes of diarrhoea in diabetes.

iii. What alternative investigations are available to establish the cause of diarrhoea in this patient?

iv. What measures can be implemented if the patient's symptoms recur?

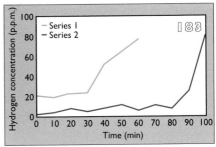

182 i. True. The salivary glands, stomach, liver, pancreas, and intestine secrete about 1500 ml, 2500 ml, 500 ml, 1500 ml and 3000 ml, respectively per day. The duodenum and jejunum (5.5 l) and ileum (2.0 l) absorb fluid to present about 1.5 l to the colon, which absorbs approximately 1.3 l. This leaves 200 ml to be excreted.
ii. True. The folds of Kerkring, villi and microvilli show an increased surface area by factors of 3, 10, and 20, respectively.
iii. False. Whereas sodium absorption in the jejunum is mainly passive, absorption through the ileum is linked to hydrogen ion secretion, and chloride absorption is linked to bicarbonate secretion. Sodium entry into the enterocyte involves an exchange for hydrogen ion. The cellular hydrogen ion originates from the hydration of CO_2, catalysed by carbonic anhydrase. Upon entry into the lumen, the hydrogen ion combines with intraluminal bicarbonate to form CO_2 and water, hence the rise in luminal pCO_2. *In vivo*, chloride ion absorption involves a bicarbonate exchange, presumably mediated by an ion-exchanger in the brush-border membrane. This carrier allows absorption of chloride ion and secretion of bicarbonate against their respective electrochemical gradients.
iv. True. Sodium absorption is accomplished by a carrier mechanism mediated by a mobile ion-exchanger. Non-electrolyte molecules such as glucose markedly stimulate sodium absorption. The apparent affinity of the carrier of sodium and glucose is greater on the luminal side of the enterocyte membrane than at the interior surface. This is probably a function of pH that is higher at the luminal surface. Thus, exchange of hydrogen for sodium ion at the interior surface may enhance glucose release into the cell, while the presence of glucose at the luminal surface may enhance carrier affinity for sodium. This characteristic forms the basis for the use of glucose-based solutions for treating of dehydrating enteritic illnesses.
v. True. Active sodium transport may be effected against steep electrochemical gradients and is stimulated by aldosterone.

183 i. A 7- to 10-day course of antibiotics for small-intestinal bacterial overgrowth.
ii. Pancreatic dysfunction; autonomic neuropathy; bacterial overgrowth syndrome; ischaemia.
iii. Culture of jejunal aspirate; small-bowel biopsy; urinary indican.
iv. Most patients require only a single course of therapy. However, antibiotic options in the event of recurrence include change of antibiotic, cyclic therapy with treatment 1 week in every 4, or failing that, continuous treatment for up to 2 months. Clonidine has been used for autonomic neuropathy since the predominant abnormality is adrenergic rather than vagal dysfunction. Cholestyramine has also been used as a treatment. Octreotide similarly has proved beneficial. Loperamide or codeine phosphate are commonly utilized as a symptomatic measure.
 Apart from diabetes, the other causes of bacterial overgrowth include fistulae, strictures, diverticula, blind loops, scleroderma and hypochlorhydria.

184 A 54-year-old woman with
rheumatoid arthritis has been
complaining of epigastric pain for 6
weeks.
i. Comment on the endoscopic
findings in the stomach (184).
ii. What diagnostic procedures are
carried out during endoscopy?
iii. What aetiological factors may be
involved in the pathogenesis of the
stomach lesion?
iv. What are the treatment options?

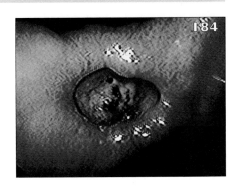

185 A 54-year-old man presented
with an effortless haematemesis. On
admission he had a pulse of 120
beats/min and a blood pressure of
70/40 mmHg. His full blood count is
given in the table.

Investigation	Result
Haemoglobin	7.6 g/dl
WBC	$12.2 \times 10^9/l$
Platelets	$75 \times 10^9/l$
MCV	104 fl

He was resuscitated and, once
stable, an upper GI endoscopy was
performed (185).
i. What is seen in 185?
ii. Are there are other sites in the GI
tract that might be similarly
affected?
iii. What causes the findings in 185?

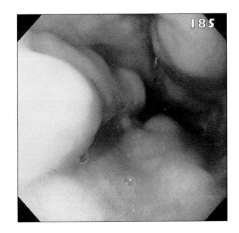

184 i. Benign gastric ulcer on the incisura.
ii. Biopsy is mandatory to exclude malignancy, plus a test for *Helicobacter pylori*.
iii. *H. pylori* infection and possible exposure to NSAIDs.
iv. If *H. pylori* is present, its eradication is essential. Triple-drug regimes – as used in the therapy of duodenal ulcer – are appropriate. If the organism is absent, NSAIDs are the likely cause and should be withdrawn if possible. Ulcer healing is then normally obtained with acid suppression therapy. Misoprostol may be added for the patient who needs to continue non-steroidals. Surgery is seldom required unless there are complications such as perforation or major haemorrhage.

It is advisable to repeat the endoscopy at 6–8 weeks to ensure healing and to confirm that an early malignancy has not been missed.

185 i. Oesophageal varices.
ii. They are most commonly recognized in the upper GI tract, particularly the oesophagus and stomach; but patients with portal hypertension may present with bleeding/melaena from the small intestine or colon.
iii. The portal vein has a very high flow rate of about 1200 ml/min, but a low resistance (normally a pressure of 7 mmHg). Varices occur due to increased portal pressure. Once portal hypertension has developed, connections between the portal and systemic circulations open up and varices may form. For portal pressure >12 mmHg, bleeding from varices is more likely.

At the oesophagogastric junction the connection between the portal and systemic circulations is extremely complex. There are four layers of venous plexi, and high portal pressures can cause these veins to dilate and alter the flow characteristics between the plexi, forming varices.

Gastric varices may form from the plexi described above and their connections with the short gastric veins. Gastric varices are often not as prominent at endoscopy as oesophageal varices because they are more deeply situated and may appear as rugal folds.

Varices in the duodenum form between afferent branches of the portal vein, such as the superior mesenteric vein and the inferior vena cava. They lie deep in the gut wall and less likely to rupture, but if they do may present with massive haematemesis or melaena.

Small-bowel varices also occur due to connections between portal and systemic circulations.

Colonic varices form from inferior mesenteric (portal circulation) and the internal iliac (systemic circulation) venous collaterals.

Rectal varices occur in collaterals between the superior haemorrhoidal vein (portal circulation) and the middle and inferior haemorrhoidal veins (systemic circulation). They must be differentiated from haemorrhoids, which are prolapses of the vascular cushions.

Varices lower down the GI tract may become more prominent once other varices, e.g. oesophageal, have been obliterated.

186 Match each of the following peptides (i–v) with their appropriate physiologic action (a–e).

i. Gastrin.
ii. Cholecystokinin (CCK).
iii. Secretin.
iv. Somatostatin.
v. Vasoactive intestinal peptide (VIP).
a. Stimulates pancreatic acinar cells, primarily to secrete trypsin, chymotrypsin and other proteins.
b. Stimulates pancreatic duct cells, primarily, to produce water and bicarbonate.
c. Stimulates intestinal fluid secretion.
d. Inhibits the release of most gastrointestinal hormones.
e. Binds to CCK-B receptors on gastric parietal cells to stimulate intrinsic factor secretion.

187 A 54-year-old woman is referred with a 30-year history of constipation. Since 20 years of age, she has used laxatives for relief of a feeling of being bloated. More recently, her bowel movements have become refractory to laxatives, which she now utilizes on a daily basis. She has also employed enemas on occasion, and reported to the emergency department the previous month when a disimpaction was performed. She has no urge to defecate and can strain for 30 minutes without producing a bowel movement. She has noticed blood on the tissue on occasion after straining. She also reports excessive stress in her life. Recently, her husband lost his job. Her dietary intake is suboptimal. She reports being afraid that eating could make her constipation worse. On examination she is thin with less than ideal weight. The left colon is palpable, containing stool. Rectally, some firm stool is present. The remainder of the examination is unremarkable. A radiograph (**187**) was taken during the work-up.

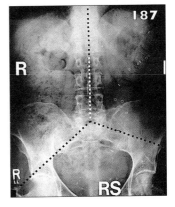

i. Which investigations are appropriate?
ii. Comment on the radiograph (**187**).
iii. What is the diagnosis?
iv. Comment on dietary and psychological issues that may be relevant.
v. Formulate a plan of treatment for this patient.

186 i. (e) Gastrin is released from G-cells located in the antrum. Gastrin stimulates acid, pepsinogen, and intrinsic factor secretion by binding to gastrin/CCK-B receptors. **ii.** (a) CCK is released from CCK cells located in the crypts and villi of the duodenum and proximal jejunum. Actions include gallbladder contraction, sphincter of Oddi relaxation, and stimulation of enzyme and protein release from pancreatic acini. **iii.** (b) Secretin is found in S-cells located primarily in the duodenum and jejunum. Release is stimulated by acidification of the duodenum and the presence of glucose, fatty acids and bile. Its main action is stimulation of water and bicarbonate secretion from pancreatic ductules. **iv.** (d) Somatostatin is found in D-cells of the pancreas, stomach and ileum, as well as nervous tissue. Somatostatin inhibits gastric acid and pepsin release, CCK/secretin-stimulated bicarbonate secretion, and insulin release. **v.** (c) VIP is located in neurones of the gut and brain. VIP stimulates secretion of pancreatic fluid and protein, and intestinal fluid. Other actions include relaxation of gastrointestinal smooth muscle and increasing intestinal blood flow.

187 i. Routine haematology and biochemical profile, thyroid function test and calcium. Sigmoidoscopy, barium enema or colonoscopy exclude a structural cause, unlikely given the very long-standing duration of her symptoms. A rectal biopsy is not often useful but may confirm melanosis coli or amyloidosis. A colon transit study may help to quantify transit time and an anorectal manometry to identify pelvic floor dysfunction. **ii.** 187 shows a colon transit study performed by ingesting a capsule containing radio-opaque markers and by taking a radiograph of the abdomen on day 6. Normally, less than 20% of markers are present. 187 shows stool with several markers distributed throughout the left colon. **iii.** Slow transit constipation (colonic inertia) may be secondary to colonic smooth muscle dysfunction, or the result of a metabolic or diffuse motor or visceral neuropathic abnormality, or laxative and cathartic abuse, and may be aggravated by dehydration and some medications. **iv.** Many patients consume insufficient fibre and may have lifestyles that promote dehydration. Surreptitious use of diuretics aggravates the constipation. Obsession with bowel movements and an intolerance of 'bloating' may lead to compulsive behaviour and depression. **v.** Withdraw medications that promote constipation, and address any metabolic problem. A diet with at least 25 g of fibre/day is instituted, and hydration optimized. A glycerine (or stimulant) suppository administered early in the morning may be useful to promote a bowel action. Endeavouring to have a bowel movement following breakfast optimizes the effects of the gastrocolic reflex. Persistent effort is important. Catharsis may be promoted by senna and osmotic laxatives. Severe cases may require polyethylene glycol for initial clearing. A colectomy may need to be considered for refractory cases, particularly in those who develop recurrent obstructive episodes or impactions.

188 A 13-year-old boy presented with a 4-month history of diarrhoea, loss of appetite and weight loss. His diarrhoea comprised small amounts of loose, offensive stool 20 to 30 times daily with no bleeding. There was no history of recent travel. He had received 7 days of ampicillin for otitis media before the onset of diarrhoea. On examination, he was obese with a body weight in excess of the 97th centile for his age. He had a subdued affect. No abnormality was found on gentle palpation of the abdomen. The stools were positive for *Clostridium difficile* toxin. An abdominal radiograph was obtained (**188**).

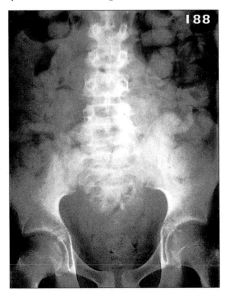

i. What is the differential diagnosis?
ii. What is the significance of the *C. difficile* in the context of the clinical story and the radiological abnormalities?
iii. How could the diagnosis have been made more easily?

189 A 23-year-old man with epigastric pain was found to have a posterior wall ulcer in the duodenal cap.
i. What investigation, performed in the endoscopy room, is shown (**189a**) and what is the significance of the result?
ii. Describe the abnormalities seen in the antral biopsy (**189b**).
iii. What are the best treatment option(s) for this patient?

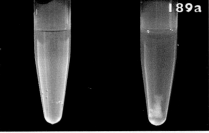

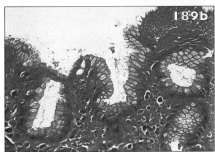

188 & 189: Answers

188 i. He has chronic constipation with overflow incontinence/diarrhoea.
ii. The differential diagnosis includes pseudomembranous colitis, inflammatory bowel disease, chronic infection/infestation, coeliac disease, laxative abuse, Hirschsprung's disease and neuroendocrine disorders. The presence of *C. difficile* toxin is strongly associated with pseudomembranous colitis, and may indicate bacterial overgrowth, but *C. difficile* is also found as a commensal in many healthy neonates and small children. Between 10% and 50% of pre-school children carry the organism without symptoms.
iii. The diagnosis in this case would have been strongly indicated by simple digital rectal examination.

189 i. This is a rapid urease test (**189a**). The pink colour change indicates the presence of the urease of *Helicobacter pylori* in this antral biopsy specimen.
ii. The histological specimen shows *H. pylori* organisms over the epithelial surface, well demonstrated by use of the Giemsa stain (**189b**); there is also an inflammatory cell infiltrate present in the mucosa.
iii. The recommended treatment is *H. pylori* eradication. The optimal regime is still a matter of controversy, but it is clear that a multi-drug regime including at least one antibiotic in combination with potent acid suppression is most likely to be successful. Penicillin sensitivity permitting, the combination of amoxycillin with metronidazole or clarithromycin and with a proton pump inhibitor, satisfies most authorities that a week's treatment should achieve a 90% eradication rate. A tetracycline can be used for those patients allergic to penicillin. Re-infection is then most unusual, and recurrence of ulceration very rare. If eradication fails, then acid suppression alone controls and heals ulcers, but with a very high relapse rate of the order of 80% within 12 months if therapy is discontinued.

190 Select the appropriate agent (A, B, C or D) for each of the following:
i. Reduces the concentration of cyclic AMP in the parietal cell.
ii. Results in an elevated serum gastrin.
iii. Interacts with the cytochrome P_{450} system in the liver.
iv. Reacts covalently with sulphhydryl groups of the cysteine residues on the extracellular surface of the alpha subunit of H^+/K^+-ATPase.
v. Associated with gastric carcinoids in humans.
A. Omeprazole.
B. Cimetidine.
C. Both omeprazole and cimetidine.
D. Neither omeprazole nor cimetidine.

191 A 66-year-old woman has recurrent episodes of severe abdominal pain, becoming increasingly frequent and more severe. The pain is generalized and requires meperidine (pethidine) to abate. She also reports episodic non-bloody diarrhoea up to six times a day, unrelated to her bouts of pain and lasting for a few days at a time, with no weight loss. In the previous week she reported occasional brown staining of her urine and passage of air bubbles on micturition. Some 10 years previously she had a hysterectomy followed by intra-cavity and external beam radiotherapy for cervical carcinoma. She has osteoarthritis and uses ibuprofen 400 mg twice daily.

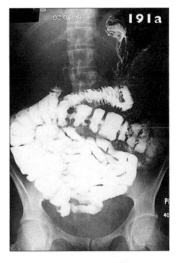

Examination is unremarkable. She undergoes colonoscopy and the ileum is entered. The small-bowel lumen is irregular and strictured with no ulceration. Histology shows no evidence of Crohn's disease. The rectal mucosa is slightly inflamed but histology is again normal. **191a** and **191b** show the appearances of a barium follow-through.
i. What is the most likely diagnosis?
ii. What other investigations are indicated?
iii. How should she be managed?

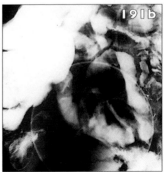

190 i. (B) Histamine binds to the parietal cell H2 receptor (H2R), which activates adenylate cyclase, increasing intracellular cyclic AMP. This induces the proton pump to secrete hydrogen ions in exchange for potassium, into the gastric lumen. H2R antagonists inhibit the binding of histamine to the H2R, reducing intracellular cyclic AMP and the secretion of acid. Gastrin and muscarinic receptors can activate the proton pump by an alternative pathway – increasing intracellular levels of calcium. Therefore, H2R blockade does not result in complete acid inhibition.
ii. (C) Since release of gastrin by antral G-cells is inhibited by a fall in gastric pH, agents that inhibit parietal cell secretion lead to an increase in plasma gastrin concentration, the magnitude of which is dependent on the degree of acid suppression. The half-life of the suppressive agent determines the duration of hypergastrinaemia. Plasma gastrin levels return to normal 2–4 weeks after discontinuation of omeprazole.
iii. (C) Both interact with hepatic cytochrome P_{450}, which therefore can inhibit the metabolism of the drug. However, this is generally not clinically significant.
iv. (A) Proton pump inhibitors are activated in the acid milieu of the parietal cell secretory canaliculus and react covalently with the sulphhydryl groups of the cysteine residues on the extracellular surface of the alpha subunit of the H^+/K^+-ATPase and inhibit the activity of the enzyme. This effectively shuts off acid secretion.
v. (D) Drugs that inhibit gastric acid secretion induce hypergastrinaemia and hyperplasia of gastric enterochromaffin-like cells. In rodent toxicity studies, administration of omeprazole resulted in the development of gastric carcinoids. Zollinger–Ellison syndrome (ZES) and pernicious anaemia (PA) are associated with a 3–5% occurrence of gastric carcinoid tumours. Neither H2R antagonists nor proton pump inhibitors have been associated with the development of gastric carcinoid tumours in humans in the absence of ZES or PA.

191 i. Radiation enterocolitis with fistula to the bladder. Other possibilities include Crohn's disease, lymphoma, intestinal TB, diverticulosis, carcinoid, and NSAID enteropathy. There were multiple small-bowel strictures and irregularities involving the distal colon.
ii. Cystography (and barium enema) to demonstrate the fistula. Breath test to establish the presence of bacterial overgrowth.
iii. Stricturing with repeated episodes of subacute obstruction is treated non-surgically unless there is an episode of significant obstruction. Fistulization to the urinary tract, however, invariably necessitates surgery. Surgery should be minimal as postoperative morbidity is high.
  Malabsorption may need to be treated, for example with antibiotics and vitamin B_{12}. Occasionally, cholestyramine is of value for bile salt diarrhoea.
  Treatment of radiation proctitis consists of topical steroid or 5-ASA medication. Mucosal telangiectasia haemorrhage is best treated with laser or bipolar cautery.

192 A 76-year-old woman recovering from aortic aneurysm repair develops left lower quadrant discomfort followed by bloody diarrhoea. She received antibiotics the week before. The haemoglobin is 10.4 g/dl; white count 15.4×10⁹/l (15400/mm³); negative stool culture; and negative stool *Clostridium difficile* toxin. A colonoscopy reveals oedema, ulceration and friability in the descending colon (192a).

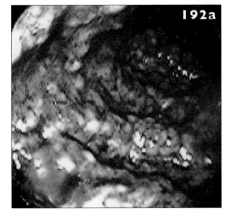

i. What is the diagnosis?
ii. Comment on the pathophysiology of this lesion.
iii. What additional confirmatory tests may be employed?
iv. Comment on treatment in this case.
v. When is surgery indicated?

193 An 8-month-old male infant has episodes of crying with flexion of the knees and hips. Two hours after an episode he has bilious vomiting. Between episodes he appears comfortable. Over time there is increasing pallor and listlessness. Physical examination reveals a soft, non-tender abdomen with a questionable mass in the right upper quadrant. An abdominal radiograph is obtained (193a).

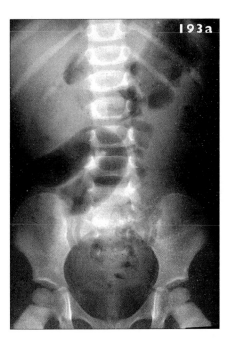

i. Describe the main abnormalities in 193a.
ii. What diagnosis is most likely?
iii. What circumstances/pathologies may precipitate this condition?
iv. How may the diagnosis be confirmed?
v. Discuss management.

192 & 193: Answers

192 i. Ischaemic colitis.
ii. The watershed region of the colon between the superior and inferior mesenteric arteries extends from the distal transverse to the sigmoid colon. This region is at increased risk for ischaemia, which may be the result of thrombosis, embolization, or non-occlusion due to hypoperfusion. A 'low-flow' state is the most common cause.

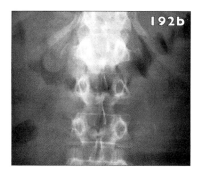

Her risk factors include age, atherosclerotic disease and aortic surgery.
iii. 'Thumbprinting' due to mucosal oedema is often seen on plain films (192b). The endoscopic appearances may be confirmed by mucosal biopsy. Mesenteric angiography is not necessary, in contradistinction to small-bowel ischaemia.
iv. Supportive treatment only. Clinical improvement generally occurs over a few days.
v. Perforation, peritonitis, excessive bleeding, and symptomatic stricturing.

193 i. Dilated loops of bowel and a paucity of air in the right lower quadrant.
ii. The history and radiograph suggest intussusception. The peak incidence is at 4–10 months.
iii. No lead point can be identified in the majority of cases. Known pathologies include swollen hypertrophied Peyer's patches, Meckel's diverticular, polyp, haemangioma, appendix and Burkitt's lymphoma.
iv. A 'currant jelly' stool may be passed. Air contrast enema is diagnostic and possibly therapeutic. Air is preferable to contrast medium because it causes less peritoneal irritation in the unlikely event of perforation, and it does not obscure later endoscopy if intussusception is absent and rectal bleeding persists.
v. Radiographic reduction (193b). The child should be observed overnight since there

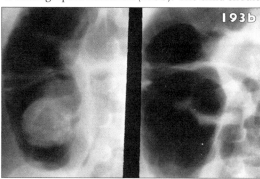

is a 3–5% recurrence rate after reduction. If radiographic reduction fails, surgery is indicated.

Index

The numbers refer to question and answer numbers, not page numbers.

Index

Index

Index

Clostridium difficile toxin, 188
Pseudo-obstruction,
acute colonic, 71
chronic intestinal, 66
Pyloric obstruction, 163
Pyloric stenosis,
hypoalbuminaemia, 181
hypokalaemia, 181
idiopathic hypertrophic, 51
Pyoderma gangrenosum, 115
inflammatory bowel disease, 141

R
Radiation,
enteritis, 50
enterocolitis, 191
proctitis, 70
Rectal ulcer syndrome, solitary, 1
Rectum,
idiopathic megarectum, 152
prolapse, 81
varices, 185
Reflux, gastro-oesophageal, 52
see also Gastro-oesophageal reflux disease (GORD)
Renal failure, 99
Rheumatoid arthritis, H. pylori and NSAIDs, 184

S
Schatski ring, 164
dysphagia, 94
hiatus hernia complication, 125
Schilling's test, vitamin B_{12} absorption, 153
Schwachman syndrome, 34
Scleroderma, intestinal, 21
Sclerosant, injection, 61
Sclerosing cholangitis, 49
primary, 28, 103
Screening, colorectal carcinoma, 84
Secretin, 186
Secretory component, gut immunity, 129
Sepsis, intra-abdominal, 166
Short bowel syndrome, renal calculi, 137
see also Crohn's disease

Small intestine,
bacterial overgrowth, 183
resection, 65
varices, 185
see also Intestine
Solitary rectal ulcer syndrome (SRUS), 1, 105
Somatostatin, 186
analogue, see Octreotide
Sprue, coeliac, 20
Stent,
oesophageal placement, 56
tumours, 56
Stool,
currant jelly, 193
osmolality, 82
Strictures,
oesophageal, 135
peptic, 170
smooth, in Crohn's disease, 12
Sucrose-isomaltase deficiency, congenital, 161
Systemic lupus erythematosus (SLE), 99
Systemic sclerosis, 130

T
Tigroid appearance, melanosis coli, 25
Trauma, vascular leak, 143
Traveller's diarrhoea, 27
E. coli, 27
Trisomy 21, see Down's syndrome
Tuberculosis, intestinal, 30, 121
Tumours,
metal stent, 56
see also Carcinoma
Typhlitis, neutropenic colitis, 112

U
Ulcer,
aphthous, 133
Crohn's disease, 15
duodenal, 111
gastric, 58
Helicobacter pylori, 85
NSAIDS, 85
oesophageal, 94
solitary rectal syndrome, 1, 105
see Peptic ulcer

Ulcerative colitis, 8, 59, 92, 115
maintenance of, remission, 29
Urease test, 189
Helicobacter pylori, 119, 189

V
Varices,
bowel, 185
colon, 185
duodenum, 185
fundic, 128
gastric, 107, 185
isolated, 128
oesophageal, 185
rectum, 185
Vasoactive intestinal peptide, 186
VIPoma,
octreotide in, 147
severe secretory diarrhoea, 151
Visceral proteins, nutritional status, 143
Vitamin A, deficiency, 165
Vitamin B_{12}
absorption, 93
Schilling's test, 153
Vomiting, cyclical syndrome, 76
Von Recklinghausen's disease, 91

W
Webs, oesophagus, 164
Whipple's disease, 95, 106

Y
Yersiniosis, 30

Z
Zinc,
copper deficiency and supplements, 142
deficiency, 108
acrodermatitis enteropathica, 108
Zollinger–Ellison syndrome, severe secretory diarrhoea, 151